WSAVA
Standards for Clinical and Histological Diagnosis of Canine and Feline Liver Disease

For Elsevier

Commissioning Editor Joyce Rodenhuis
Development Editor Rita Demetriou-Swanwick
Project Manager Caroline Horton/Nancy Arnott
Designer Andy Chapman
Illustrations Manager Bruce Hogarth

WSAVA Standards for Clinical and Histological Diagnosis of Canine and Feline Liver Disease

WSAVA Liver Standardization Group

Jan Rothuizen

Susan E. Bunch

Jenny A. Charles

John M. Cullen

Valeer J. Desmet

Viktor Szatmári

David C. Twedt

Ted S. G. A. M. van den Ingh

Tom Van Winkle

Robert J. Washabau

Foreword by Claudio Brovida and Hein Meyer

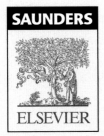

SAUNDERS

ELSEVIER

EDINBURGH   LONDON   NEW YORK   OXFORD   PHILADELPHIA   ST LOUIS   SYDNEY   TORONTO   2006

SAUNDERS
ELSEVIER

© 2006, Elsevier Limited. All rights reserved.

No part of this publication may be reproduced, stored in a retrieval system, or transmitted in any form or by any means, electronic, mechanical, photocopying, recording or otherwise, without the prior permission of the Publishers. Permissions may be sought directly from Elsevier's Health Sciences Rights Department, 1600 John F. Kennedy Boulevard, Suite 1800, Philadelphia, PA 19103-2899, USA: phone: (+1) 215 239 3804; fax: (+1) 215 239 3805; or, e-mail: *healthpermissions@elsevier.com*. You may also complete your request on-line via the Elsevier homepage (http://www.elsevier.com), by selecting 'Support and contact' and then 'Copyright and Permission'.

First published 2006

ISBN-10: 0-7020-2791-X
ISBN-13: 978-0-7020-2791-8

British Library Cataloguing in Publication Data
A catalogue record for this book is available from the British Library

Library of Congress Cataloging in Publication Data
A catalog record for this book is available from the Library of Congress

Notice
Knowledge and best practice in this field are constantly changing. As new research and experience broaden our knowledge, changes in practice, treatment and drug therapy may become necessary or appropriate. Readers are advised to check the most current information provided (i) on procedures featured or (ii) by the manufacturer of each product to be administered, to verify the recommended dose or formula, the method and duration of administration, and contraindications. It is the responsibility of the practitioner, relying on their own experience and knowledge of the patient, to make diagnoses, to determine dosages and the best treatment for each individual patient, and to take all appropriate safety precautions. To the fullest extent of the law, neither the Publisher nor the Authors assumes any liability for any injury and/or damage to persons or property arising out or related to any use of the material contained in this book.

The Publisher

Working together to grow
libraries in developing countries

www.elsevier.com | www.bookaid.org | www.sabre.org

ELSEVIER   BOOK AID
            International   Sabre Foundation

The publisher's policy is to use **paper manufactured from sustainable forests**

Printed in Spain

Contents

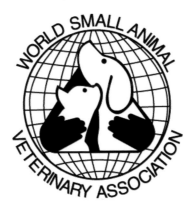

WSAVA Liver Standardization Group

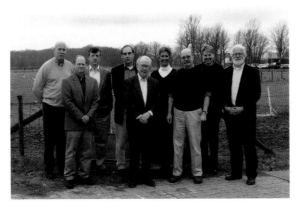

The WSAVA Liver Standardization Group during one of the working meetings, early spring 2003 in Utrecht. Left to right: Ted van den Ingh, David Twedt, John Cullen, Jan Rothuizen, Valeer Desmet, Susan Bunch, Tom Van Winkle, Jenny Charles, Robert Washabau. Absent: Viktor Szatmári.

Preface and acknowledgements

Jan Rothuizen

This book is the result of the joint efforts of many people and it has been written for use by those working in veterinary practice, by veterinary pathologists, and by scientists in academia.

This is the first world standard for the definition and nomenclature of diseases in small animal medicine, and the authors hope this joint international initiative will be the start of many comparable efforts to bring veterinarians from all over the world to consensus. Bearing in mind that standards will need to be updated, we expect that within 3 to 4 years, it will be necessary to publish an updated world standard for the diagnosis of liver diseases. The authors of this book invite readers to support this standardization by supplying them with new information that may lead to the definition of new diseases or re-definition of existing ones. The authors are also open to any comment on the content of this book.

The group owes a special word of gratitude to those who have made this book possible. First of all, to Dr Claudio Brovida, President of the WSAVA until October 2002, who had the vision to help this book come to fruition, and in the process, hopefully to set the stage for world-wide professional cooperation in many other areas of veterinary medicine. The veterinary world owes Claudio lasting recognition for his vision, and our specialist group feels it has been a privilege to have been able to complete the first standardization exercise with his help. The authors are glad that Brovida keeps representing the board, because he has initiated the standardization iniative. The continuous setting and updating of world standards has become a key activity of the WSAVA which will enable our group to update the present book. Thanks also go to a special member of the Liver Standardization Group, Professor Valeer Desmet from the Medical School of Leuven, Belgium. Professor Desmet has been engaged with all the human liver standardization exercises over the past 30 years or more, and he can really be considered to be one of the co-founders of modern human liver pathology. The presence of such a great expert in our group has been, and will remain to be, crucially stimulating. He is a pure scientist who is open to any scientific argument, and he takes an active part in the often sharp, but never personal or unfriendly debates about the issues under discussion. It is a strength of the group that it was possible for arguments to be open, direct, and always scientific; and when the veterinarians could not reach agreement it was always the expert in human pathology who helped to find the way out. We as veterinarians cannot overestimate the value of his contribution, which he gave freely, without any personal remuneration.

Foreword

The aim of the WSAVA is to promote continuing education and to enhance standards of veterinary education throughout the world. The hepatic standardization project developed as a concept in July 2000 following discussions with Dr Jan Rothuizen of the Utrecht Veterinary School about a widespread disparity in the diagnostic reporting of the pathology of liver disease. It was a strange fact that in this modern world, international experts on the five continents used differing terminologies to describe the pathological changes taking place in the liver.

An international committee of world-renowned specialists was convened and the result is seen in this publication which will contribute enormously to the diagnosis of hepatic disease, and it is hoped, become the standard subject text of the future.

The WSAVA has worked closely with Hill's Pet Nutrition on many projects and has been fortunate to have had, once again, the full support of this company in seeing this 2-year project to completion. The enrichment and lenghtening of the special relationships between people and pets is the mission statement of Hill's Pet Nutrition and this project has contributed to both this mission statement and to knowledge and welfare throughout the veterinary world.

This initiative has been so well received by veterinary educators that it has been followed by a second project working with international gastroenterologists who will be reporting at the Prague WSAVA Congress in 2006 on the standardization of the nomenclature of the pathology of gastrointestinal disease.

Claudio Brovida DVM

Past president, WSAVA

Hein Meyer DVM, PhD, Dipl-ECVIM Director, Hill's Pet Nutrition, Inc.

Chapter **1**

Introduction – background, aims and methods

Jan Rothuizen

This book is for use in veterinary practice and pathology as an aid in making and understanding the diagnosis of all liver diseases known to date, in dogs and cats. It is also meant to be a guide for the veterinary profession in the standardized diagnostic approach and nomenclature of liver diseases.

BACKGROUND

The diagnosis of liver diseases depends on the interpretation of the outcome of a number of examinations. Central to the diagnostic process is the interpretation of the liver histology examination, and for most liver diseases, this is the essential step in making a good diagnosis. Clinicians and pathologists, therefore, need to cooperate closely in order to understand each other's input in making decisions about the true diagnosis.

In general, and certainly also in the histopathological evaluation of liver disorders, there tends to be a large variation in the interpretation of a particular tissue by different pathologists. Samples from one case may produce up to six different diagnoses when evaluated by ten pathologists. Such large interobserver variations do also exist for many other observations made during the diagnostic process. However, since the histopathological evaluation is critical for the diagnosis of liver diseases, this aspect is a cornerstone of our attempt to set up a world standard for diagnostic criteria of liver diseases of companion animals.

The apparent lack of standard criteria for defining the diagnosis has had serious consequences.

Firstly, in everyday practice there must have been many cases in which the diagnosis was not correct, with the result that clinicians have treated many dogs and cats with the wrong medication. Many veterinarians have the impression that liver diseases are difficult to treat, but this is in fact not true for the vast majority of these diseases. A solid diagnosis might usually be followed by successful therapy, but it may also make clear that there is no treatment possible. A solid diagnosis is therefore the basis for all logical and evidence-based veterinary interventions.

Secondly, on reading the scientific literature it becomes clear that reports on a particular disease cannot be compared with reports on the same disease in other publications, simply because the criteria are different; it is also not unusual to find that different diseases are reported under the same name. This may make it very hard to compare the results and conclusions of one publication with those of another and such confusion hinders the potential progress of veterinary medicine because it takes much time and many studies before the truth becomes apparent and generally accepted. Good comparability of different publications on a particular disease is not the only profit to be gained. The development of rationally validated treatments has been largely hampered by the lack of solid diagnostic criteria. When reviewing the literature, it is apparent that there are very few, if any, medications of liver diseases that have been tested in double-blind, placebo-controlled studies. Such studies are required to make decisions about the best treatment regimes for diseases, and to decide about the added value of newly developed treatments in the future. Given the caseload of most specialized clinics, controlled studies of the therapeutic effect of drugs can only be performed during a reasonable time span with the cooperation of different centers in each study (multicenter studies). It is now time to make progress in this direction, but it is only possible when different participating centers can use solid and undisputed diagnostic criteria.

Thirdly, confusion has increased even further owing to the fact that certain diseases have been given more than one name. There has been insufficient reference to the existing literature and lack of scientific discussion to prevent this happening, with the result that differences in nomenclature seem to have occurred between the different continents. Because the standardization process in this book has been performed by specialists from all over the world, it has been possible, where applicable, to propose one standard name where different names exist for one disease.

Examination

Pathomorphological examination is important, but it is only part of the diagnostic process for liver diseases. One of the most important advances in the past decade has been the complete incorporation of ultrasonography into veterinary medicine; and certainly for the diagnostic process of liver diseases, ultrasound examination has become an indispensable tool. The generally accepted parameters for evaluation by ultrasonography are summarized in Chapter 2 along with techniques for liver biopsy. Although the Liver Study Group has primarily focused on the role of pathological interpretation and its interaction with clinical hepatology including clinical pathology, it was felt that limiting evaluation to this approach in this way would give rise to incomplete standards for the diagnosis of all other diseases. In the vascular liver diseases, particularly, ultrasonographic examination is an essential cornerstone in combination with clinical pathological and histological examination; therefore, Dr Viktor Szatmári (Universtity of Utrecht), who had developed and published standard protocols for ultasonographic evaluation of vascular liver diseases, was invited to write a chapter on this subject. For these diseases, standard protocols are described in Chapter 3, which permits the location of portosystemic shunts and other vascular changes with a large degree of certainty.

Hematological and biochemical examinations are an integral part of the diagnostic process for liver diseases. However, most of these examinations are not a decisive factor in the diagnosis of a liver disease, but serve only to differentiate liver disease from other diseases with similar symptoms and signs. As soon as the presence of a liver disease has been demonstrated (e.g. by elevated liver enzymes or bile acids in plasma, or clinical icterus) the role of the blood examination in making a decision on the diagnosis is very weak for most liver diseases, except in the vascular disorders. Therefore the reader will find little information about blood examinations that is not essential in the diagnostic process.

This book starts at the point where the presence of a liver disease is apparent through the finding of elevated plasma enzymes, bile acids, or the presence of icterus.

AIMS

The main aim of this book is to describe world-wide-accepted standards and criteria for the diagnosis of all known liver diseases of dogs and cats. Pathologists and clinicians will find well-defined histological diagnostic criteria and precise definitions of chronicity stages. The variations with which diseases may present are described and examples are given. In addition, unified nomenclature is proposed if a disease has been given different names in the past; and clearly descriptive names are proposed. The necessary combination of diagnostic methods and their relative roles is given in tables, so that the reader will have an immediate review of the essentials of the diagnostic process. The reader will find all the relevant technical details about the diagnostic procedures used by clinicians, pathologists, and ultrasonographers.

We have attempted to give relevant pictures of all liver diseases and their variations in dogs and cats.

METHODS

The liver study group

In cooperation with and under the auspices of the Board of the World Small Animal Veterinary Association (WSAVA), an international Liver Standardization Group was formed, consisting of internationally recognized scientists in hepatogastroenterology. Pathologists who specialize in the liver and expert clinicians were invited from the USA to become part of the group, Europe, and Australia. In addition, one of the top human liver pathologists was invited as an independent back-up and to help in making decisions during the course

of debate on difficult topics. The Liver Standardization Group was not only formed under the auspices of the WSAVA, but also supported by the boards of the European and American Colleges of Veterinary Internal Medicine (ECVIM and ACVIM). The expert group was composed as follows:

Dr S. Bunch (USA), clinical hepatologist (North Carolina State University); Dr J. A. Charles (Australia), liver pathologist (University of Melbourne); Dr J. Cullen (USA), liver pathologist (North Carolina State Univesity); Dr V. J. Desmet (Belgium, Europe), human liver pathologist (University of Leuven); Dr T. S. G. A. M. van den Ingh (Netherlands, Europe), liver pathologist (University of Utrecht); Dr T. Van Winkle (USA), liver pathologist (University of Pennsylvania); Dr D. C. Twedt (USA), clinical hepatologist (Colorado State University); Dr R. J. Washabau (USA), gastroenterologist/hepatologist (University of Minnesota); Dr J. Rothuizen (Netherlands, Europe), clinical hepatologist, coordinator of the group (University of Utrecht).

This group has met twice a year over a 3-year period. Each year there was a meeting during the American ACVIM forum and one during the European ECVIM congress. The agreements on standardization reached in the previous period were presented at the specialist meetings of the two congresses, so that the reactions of the veterinary specialists in the field could be incorporated in the final standards developed. The pathologists of the group have also presented the consensus diagnostic criteria at the American and European Veterinary Pathology congresses.

The liver diseases were divided into four groups:

1. Vascular liver disorders
2. Biliary tract disorders
3. Parenchymal disorders including stellate cells and Kupffer cells
4. Neoplasia.

An exhaustive list was made of all liver diseases in the four groups, and cases were collected in all centers participating in the standardization group. In several publications, veterinarians from practice or academia were also invited to submit samples or other contributions.

Two months before the meeting the pathologists had exchanged representative samples of tissue of all these diseases. All veterinary pathologists had selected three cases of each of the diseases of which they had paraffin-embedded liver tissue available. They selected those cases based on their feeling that they were representative for the disease. If appropriate, they also selected representative cases of acute, subacute, and chronic stages, or mild, moderate, and severe stages. Since there should be the possibility for each pathologist to make specific stains of liver slides, each participating center submitted four unstained slices of each selected tissue. Each pathologist thus possessed an identical set of slides of all diseases (ten or more cases per disease), so that it was possible to evaluate them in the months before the meeting, and to start to discuss them over the telephone and e-mail in preparation for the meeting. This culminated in the production of hundreds of slides by all pathologists.

During the meeting the members of the Liver Standardization Group evaluated all slides and the relevant clinical aspects of the diseases. Although there was a lot of discussion about the cases, it was not hard to reach consensus. A smaller selection was made from all slides that were considered to represent the typical features for all diseases. Ted van den Ingh has made a collection of the typical slides for all diseases for publication in this book.

Chapter 2

Sampling and handling of liver tissue

Jan Rothuizen, Valeer J. Desmet,
Ted S. G. A. M. van den Ingh, David C. Twedt,
Susan E. Bunch, Robert J. Washabau

CHAPTER CONTENTS

MAKING A DIAGNOSIS IS CLINICOPATHOLOGICAL TEAMWORK

The diagnosis of most liver diseases depends essentially on histopathological examination of liver tissue. This is especially the case for parenchymal liver diseases, many biliary tract diseases, and tumors of the liver or biliary tract. The diagnosis of circulatory liver diseases depends largely on combined information obtained with laboratory examination, ultrasonography, and histopathological evaluation. The clinician has to combine the parts of the puzzle to make the diagnosis. To date, ultrasonography plays the central role in diagnosis of most circulatory liver diseases.[1,2] Standard protocols for ultrasonographic detection of vascular liver disorders are given in Chapter 3.

Compared to human medicine, liver histopathology in veterinary medicine is even more important. The most evident example is hepatitis, which is a frequent disease in both humans and dogs. However, veterinarians do not (yet) know the etiology of most forms and depend completely on careful pathological characterization, whereas in humankind most forms are caused by known viruses which can be diagnosed using serological tests. In accordance with the essential role of histopathology in the diagnosis of liver diseases of companion animals, this book is largely devoted to the careful description of the histopathological diagnostic criteria of canine and feline liver diseases. However, the diagnosis is always based on the interactions between the clinician, the pathologist, the ultrasonographer, and sometimes other specialists.

The clinician should supply the pathologist with all the relevant clinical information. It is also very important that the clinician understands the possibilities and limitations of various tissue sampling techniques; it is obvious that focal lesions may be missed by taking random samples. Before taking a biopsy of any kind the clinician should verify whether the lesions are diffuse or local; this can usually be determined with ultrasonography. Local abnormalities should be sampled under ultrasound guidance in order to make sure the tissue is obtained from the abnormal area. It is not always good to sample the center of the lesion; for example, hepatocellular neoplasms tend to become very large and may develop central necrosis. Such lesions are best sampled in the peripheral regions. If the liver is diffusely affected (most liver diseases) the tissue samples may be obtained from random sites. In any case, liver biopsies should be as representative as possible. Two or three different samples are much better than one. One good core needle biopsy represents only 150000th of the organ. The liver is composed of liver lobules (acini), and it is important for the pathologist to be able to assess all zones of the micro-architecture including the portal (acinus zone 1) as well as centrolobular (zone 3) areas. Two well-taken needle biopsies usually contain several representations of the micro-architecture, which is enough to permit reliable evaluation.[3,4] However, one should be aware that exceptions might occur. In the case of macronodular cirrhosis, a puncture might miss the inflammatory and fibrotic areas and come up with only the hyperplastic tissue.

It is also important for the clinician to know that the pathologist may need different approaches. This is often only possible when the tissue is collected appropriately. For most approaches tissue is fixed in 10% neutral buffered formalin. However, electron microscopy requires specific fixation, and many procedures such as immunohistochemisty, in situ hybridization, and reverse transcriptase-polymerase chain reaction ((RT)-PCR) are best performed on snap-frozen tissue. If there is doubt it is useful to consult the pathologist about the storage or fixation technique before taking the tissue samples, so that maximum gain can be obtained from the collected samples. The general rules for tissue sample handling are summarized later in this chapter.

Diagnosis of liver diseases is teamwork. Cooperation between different specialists, who mutually understand each other's requirements and possibilities, is necessary for the best possible results. The clinicopathological team is central in this joint effort.

PATIENT PREPARATION

Fasting

It is important to have the patient fasted for about 12 hours. The stomach covers the visceral surface of the liver and a full stomach may prevent approach to the liver. Moreover, the liver stores glycogen according to the daily fluctuations in carbohydrate intake. It is easier to interpret the glycogen amount in the hepatocytes when animals are compared in a similar fasting condition. Nonetheless, nausea and decreased appetite are regular symptoms in hepatobiliary diseases so that long-term feeding conditions are variable by nature. Another reason for keeping the animal fasted before liver tissue sampling is that some dogs and most cats require anesthesia.

Blood coagulation testing

Blood coagulation testing is very important before taking a liver biopsy, and should be performed shortly beforehand because coagulation parameters may change quickly in such patients; therefore blood for the coagulation tests should not be sampled more than 24 hours before taking the biopsy. Presently, this is the most difficult requirement to meet in private practice, now that ultrasound-guided biopsy techniques have become generally available. The possible reasons for abnormal coagulation due to hepatobiliary diseases are reduced production of clotting factors, inadequate intestinal resorption of vitamin K, and diffuse intravascular coagulation (DIC). All of these processes may play a role. The majority of dogs with liver disease have one or more abnormal coagulation tests.[5-8] Diseases with severe cholestasis may lead to vitamin K deficiency reflected by prolonged prothrombin time and increased PIVKAs (proteins induced by vitamin K absence); in diseases with severely reduced hepatic protein production, such as cirrhosis, inadequate production of clotting factors may be most prominent; in diseases characterized by diffuse necrosis of the liver (hepatitis, malignant lymphoma) which may activate the clotting cascade, DIC is likely to be the major cause. It is generally advised to measure prothrombin time (PTT), activated thromboplastin time (APTT), and platelet count.[5-9] Liver biopsy should then be avoided in case of severe coagulopathy. Note that there is no published information indicating beyond which limits of abnormal coagulation tests it becomes unsafe to take liver biopsies. We have found, empirically, that fibrinogen is the most critical indicator, and that reductions below 50% of the lower 95% reference level (1 g/L) were contraindications for taking a biopsy. Experience has taught us that complications due to prolonged bleeding occurred frequently below this level, and that complications could not be predicted with prolonged PTT or APTT or with reduced thrombocyte count. Prospective application of this single criterion to 1000 dogs in the Companion Animal Clinic of Utrecht University resulted in the exclusion of 6% of the dogs from biopsy. Of the other 94% only three cases developed clinically detectable hemorrhage that was never fatal; one case required blood transfusion. Nearly all dogs of the 6% group with very low fibrinogen proved to have hepatitis or diffuse neoplastic liver disease. Fibrinogen had increased to above the critical level after 1 week of treatment with prednisolone in > 90% of the dogs with hepatitis so that a liver tissue sample could be taken by then. In cats with liver disease, the majority had one or more clotting abnormalities, predominantly caused by vitamin K deficiency and which responded to vitamin K1 administration.[10,11] Again, there is no information available about the exact limits beyond which liver biopsy sampling is contraindicated. In our experience at least a doubling of the PTT can be tolerated. Based on the literature it may be advisable to pretreat cats with prolonged PTT with vitamin K1 parenterally. If blood clotting parameters (fibrinogen, PTT) are within the reference range there is no need to check for post-biopsy bleeding with ultrasonogra-

phy. In cases with borderline coagulation it is safe to have fresh frozen plasma available and evaluate bleeding after 30–60 min with ultrasonography. Fresh frozen plasma can also be given as preventive treatment 2 hours prior to the procedure.

Ultrasound examination

Ultrasound examination of the abdominal cavity, focusing on the liver, biliary tract and portal vein, is an essential preparation before liver tissue is sampled. Systematic evaluation is required of:

1. The size of the liver
2. The presence of local changes or a diffusely even architecture
3. Diameter and wall thickness of extrahepatic and intrahepatic bile ducts
4. The gall bladder
5. Vascular changes, especially of the portal vein
6. The presence of free abdominal fluid.

These criteria are relevant for the preparation of tissue sampling. A very small liver may be hard to approach, and if only an intercostal approach is possible it may be advisable to anesthetize the animal. If the liver is enlarged it is important to rule out severe congestion, which is a contraindication for tissue sampling and in itself is not a good indication for taking a biopsy. Local changes should be sampled with ultrasound guidance, whereas diffuse changes can be sampled randomly. Local changes such as mucocele may have a very typical echo-structure. If the liver structure is diffusely irregular it is advisable to take more samples (at least three) in order to represent the changes as well as possible. The bile ducts may be distended due to extrahepatic bile duct obstruction or cholangitis (especially in cats). Distension of the gall bladder is not a sign of common bile duct obstruction. In the case of a dilated common bile duct, ultrasonographic evaluation of the pancreas, duodenal wall, and region of Vater's papilla may reveal the cause of an obstruction, which is already diagnostic. Otherwise a liver biopsy is required; in cats this is the only way to distinguish cholangitis from obstruction. Calcifications are usually located in the wall of the bile ducts and may indicate chronic inflammation, tumor or cystic lesions arising from the biliary tree. The gall bladder may contain bile stones, or have a thickened and sometimes edematous wall; an abnormal wall of the gall bladder is an indication for fine needle aspiration of bile for cytology and culture. Vascular diseases of the portal vein usually lead to a typical and uniform histological pattern, and ultrasonography is essential to diagnose several changes such as congenital portosystemic shunts or arteriovenous fistulas (see Ch. 3); some vascular diseases require the combination of ultrasonography and histology of the liver. The presence of free abdominal fluid often makes penetration of the liver with the puncture needle harder, especially because the liver is much firmer than normal in many cases so that the liver floats away from the needle when punctured. In such cases it may be necessary to use an automatic biopsy gun. In the presence of dilation of the bile ducts it is very important to take care to avoid the bile ducts because puncturing these with a thick needle may lead to a severe vagal reaction with hypotension and shock.

Anesthesia

The last aspect of patient preparation is the required form of anesthesia. For cats it is always recommended to give general anesthesia as very few cats are sufficiently cooperative to allow the use of local anesthesia. In dogs, however, as a rule, liver biopsy can be taken under local anesthesia.[12] It is only in very rare uncooperative dogs or when the liver is so small that an intercostal approach[13] is required that it may be better to give general anesthesia. General anesthesia in itself is a risk factor when liver functions are severely impaired. Local anesthesia (with lidocaine) includes the skin, subcutis and abdominal wall. The liver is completely painless if the larger bile ducts are avoided.

HANDLING THE LIVER TISSUE[3,4]

It is important to treat the tissue samples appropriately in order to provide the pathologist with the best possible material. The following guidelines may be helpful:

1. Verify the quality of the tissue. The aim is to have at least two, and preferably three pieces of tissue. Core needle or true cut biopsies should be unfragmented and preferably 2 cm in length. Thick pieces of tissue obtained surgically can best be sliced into 2–3 mm thick portions in order to let the fixative penetrate adequately.

2. Quick fixation is essential. The tissue should be put into the fixative within 2 min. The routine fixative is 10% neutral buffered formalin. For fixation time see guideline 4.

3. Think in advance about the specific questions to be answered. It may be necessary to carry out electron microscopy, specific stains for metabolic diseases, etc. In such cases it is best to contact the pathologist to discuss the preferred fixatives.

4. For enzyme histochemistry, immunohistochemistry or in situ hybridization it is not always possible to use formalin-fixed tissue. Instead, it may be necessary to use cryostat sections. For this, it is important to snap-freeze the tissue in such a way that the architecture is not disturbed by crystal formation. Such tissues should be frozen in isopentane, which has been precooled in liquid nitrogen. After this process the tissue can be stored in the freezer at −70°C. Such snap-frozen tissues can also be used for (quantitative) RT-PCR studies. Freezing the tissue in a freezer is too slow a process as it results in severe atrefacts created by large ice crystals that form during freezing.

5. If only ribonucleic acid (RNA) or deoxyribonucleic acid (DNA) are to be preserved, without the need to recognize the architecture of the tissue, it is adequate to put the tissue in a cryo-vial and to freeze it directly in liquid nitrogen; long-term storage is then possible in the freezer at −70°C. For long-term preservation of RNA it can best be frozen submerged in a preservant such as RNA-later. This procedure should be used for molecular techniques on the DNA/RNA of the sampled tissue, such as (quantitative) PCR, miroarray assays, quantitative analysis of proteins, etc.

6. For quantitative measurement of metals in liver, such as copper, avoid saline, because neutron activation analysis for the measurement of small amounts in biopsy samples is disturbed by the presence of sodium. Tissue should be sampled in a metal-free plastic container and freeze-

dried; thereafter closed containers can be stored at room temperature.

7. Do not let the sample dry. Take care of quick procedures and avoid putting the tissue on a paper or cloth towel. Use a saline-moistened plastic sheet instead.
8. Take care that the tissue does not fragment during transport. A tube half filled with fixative will shake and cause fragmentation of the tissue; therefore fill the tube completely with fixative so that the sample is not shaken.
9. Bacterial infections of the liver are very rare so there is no indication for routine culture of liver samples.[14,15] Sampling for culturing is indicated only when bacterial infection is likely, based on histological examination or other findings (phlegmona seen with ultrasound or radiography).

LIVER BIOPSY TECHNIQUES; ADVANTAGES, DISADVANTAGES, RECOMMENDATIONS

There are several techniques for obtaining liver tissue for examination and each has advantages and disadvantages. There is no absolute recommendation for the use of one specific method; it is, however, important to understand the possibilities and limitations and to choose the best method under the given circumstances. All biopsies should, of course, be performed under sterile conditions (hair clipping, washing, disinfection).

NEEDLE BIOPSY DEVICES

Needle biopsy can be obtained with three needle types:[3,4,9,12–14,16–18]

1. Histological biopsies can be obtained with a cutting needle which entraps the tissue after cutting it off. The original needle was the Vim-Silvermann needle, which was later replaced by the True-cut needle.
2. Tissue can be obtained by aspiration (with saline) using a syringe attached to the needle. This technique was first reported by Menghini and is still referred to as the Menghini technique.
3. Isolated cells for cytological examination are obtained with a fine needle by aspiration with an empty syringe which is attached to the needle.

True-cut needles

True-cut needles have an inner needle with a 2 cm long indentation, which is first inserted into the liver so that the tissue can fall into the indentation. The outer needle with a cutting edge is then inserted over the inner needle so that the tissue is sliced off, after which the entire instrument is withdrawn. True-cut needles have sharp tips that can easily penetrate different structures, and should therefore only be used under ultrasound guidance or direct vision such as during surgery. True-cut needles come in three types: manual, semi-automatic and for use in a biopsy-gun (Fig. 2.1).

Figure 2.1 An example of an automatic True-cut needle gun with a 14 G needle (top), a semi-automatic 16 G True-cut needle which can be used in cats (middle), and a 14 G Menghini needle attached to a disposable syringe filled with saline. The True-cut needles are disposable and the Menghini needle is re-usable.

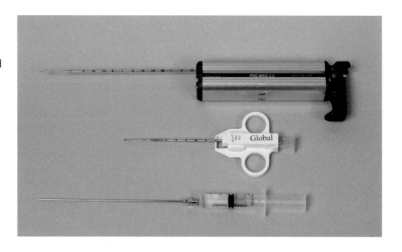

Semi-automatic needles are the most expensive but are very easy to use; these needles are recommended for use with cats. Manual devices are more difficult to control and their handling takes more time, which means that there is more of a chance of inducing rupture of the liver lobe during respiratory excursions. The biopsy gun is expensive, but the gun needles are cheap, which is attractive for centers where biopsies are routinely taken.

An advantage of the True-cut gun is that the process is so quick that a small firm fibrotic liver moving freely in ascites cannot escape. In such cases it may be impossible to obtain samples with other techniques. In general, True-cut needles produce nice unfragmented pieces of tissue in all cases. A disadvantage is that 50% of the lumen of the external needle is filled with the inner needle; the same diameter Menghini needle produces biopsies that are twice as large.[12] A special note should be made about the use of biopsy gun devices in cats. We have used a gun with True-cut needles for cats, and have experienced a remarkably high percentage of (often fatal) cases of vagal shock reaction within 15–30 min after taking the biopsies. After a few months we made the connection between this sudden rise in complication rate (from 0.05 to 25%) and the change in approach, and replaced the gun needles with much more gentle semi-automatic True-cut devices. Ever since, the complication rate has fallen to usual figures, so that we concluded that cats, unlike dogs and human patients, do not tolerate the sudden shock wave brought about by the gun device.

In summary, True-cut needles should be used under ultrasound guidance, which is the best approach for less experienced samplers. The semi-automatic needles are easiest to handle, and are recommended for cats. True-cut gun devices are superior in sampling fibrotic tissue and cheap when biopsies are taken routinely; they should however be avoided in cats.

The Menghini aspiration needle

Handling the Menghini aspiration needle is quite different from handling True-cut needles. This needle has a tip with a blunt angle, which can penetrate soft tissues such as the liver but not firm tissues.[12] The tip of the needle can be used to 'palpate' the tissues in front, and with enough experience, it is easy to locate the liver and avoid structures such as the intestines, stomach and diaphragm. This needle is used for the 'blind' biopsy technique, without ultrasound guidance (Fig. 2.2). It is therefore not possible to perform guided sampling of focal lesions so that this technique is only applicable if the liver is diffusely affected. This applies to most liver diseases, but should first be verified by ultrasonography. The Menghini technique is also suitable for follow-up

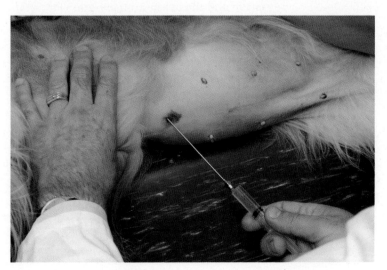

Figure 2.2 Position of a dog during the Menghini biopsy procedure. The dog is locally anesthetized, in right lateral recumbancy with the abdominal wall at the edge of the table. The needle is entered into the abdominal cavity via a midline incision 2–3 cm caudal to the xyphoid.

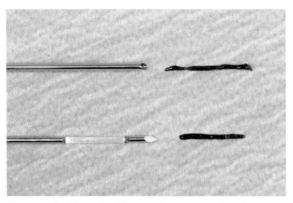

Figure 2.3 Tips of a Menghini needle (top) and a True-cut needle (bottom) with typical biopsy samples obtained with these needles. Both needles are 14 Gauge (G) and the length of the True-cut sample is 2 cm. In cross-section the shape of a True-cut sample is half-circular, whereas the Menghini needle exploits the full diameter of the needle.

biopsies in the evaluation of diffuse liver diseases such as hepatitis, where ultrasonography is not required. This blind technique should not be used in the case of distended bile ducts. It is also not advisable for cats because it requires much experience to be sure to avoid critical structures in small animals without control by vision. The Menghini technique, however, also has distinct advantages which makes it attractive for specialized clinics with a large caseload and in research conditions. The method is much cheaper than other methods because no ultrasonography is required and Menghini cannulas can be re-used many times. In experienced hands the Menghini technique is also quicker than any other system. The samples are twice as big as those obtained with comparable diameter True-cut needles because the entire lumen is used to capture the sample (Fig. 2.3).

The percutaneous blind Menghini technique is performed as follows. As for True-cut biopsies, only local anesthesia is required (skin, subcutis, abdominal wall). Because the gallbladder lies on the right side, the biopsy is obtained from the left lateral liver lobe to prevent rupture of the gallbladder and also of large blood vessels and bile ducts in the hilus. The left lateral liver lobe is by far the biggest and with some experience it is easy to locate. For dogs the best needle size is 18 cm

long and 14 gauge (G) for medium and large sized dogs, and 16 G for small dogs. The typical biopsy weight is 20–30 mg. With the dog lying on its right side and the abdominal wall at the edge of the table, the Menghini needle is introduced in the median line 1–2 cm behind the xiphoid process. After disinfection of the skin and local injection of a few mL of lidocaine, a small incision through the abdominal wall is made with a surgical blade (no. 11), to permit introduction of the Menghini cannula. The needle is attached to a saline-filled disposable syringe of 5 mL, which is used to aspirate tissue while forwarding the needle into the liver. The bluntly tipped needle is used to carefully 'palpate' intraabdominal structures without immediately penetrating them. The left lateral liver lobe should be located with certainty while avoiding other structures such as the stomach (which is painful) or the diaphragm. The dog should be fasted so that the stomach can easily be avoided. Before reaching these structures the needle is forwarded through the falciform ligament and then fat is flushed out of the cannula with some saline. 'Palpation' of the liver with the needle tip requires experience; it is within immediate reach in brachycephalic breeds with a wide thorax and more cranial in racing dog types. The tip of the needle is forwarded 0.5–1.0 cm into the liver and then further under gentle aspiration for another 2–3 cm. This brings a 2–3 cm core sample into the needle. In a continuous movement the needle is then withdrawn under permanent aspiration to retain the tissue in the needle. The Menghini needle contains a mandrin 3 cm shorter than the needle, which prevents liver tissue being aspirated and fragmented in the syringe.

Fine needle aspiration

Fine needle aspiration is performed with a 20–22 G needle.[19,20] A disposable injection needle is usually sufficient, but for deep lesions longer needles may be required. The procedure is identical to that used for any other structure punctured for cytological examination. The main difference with histological biopsies obtained by wide bore needles, forceps or surgery is that cells are obtained without the histological context. The aspirate is put on a mounting glass and dried. Routine staining is with May-Grünwald-Giemsa, but it is also possible to use specific staining methods, e.g. with rubeanic acid or rhodanine for intracellular copper granules. Fine needle puncture is usually performed under ultrasound guidance in order to sample cells from a focal lesion. However, it is also possible to obtain 'blind' samples by puncturing the liver in the 10th intercostal space at the level of the connection of rib to rib-cartilage. Cytology of the liver is not suitable for any disease in which the histological structure is required for proper judgement. This applies to the vast majority of liver diseases. Fine needle aspiration is useful only if it is possible for the diagnosis to be made in single isolated cells. This applies to the identification of tumor cells from a local lesion, or changes which are diffusely present in all hepatocytes such as steatosis (fatty liver) or steroid hepatopathy. Possible underlying liver pathology will, however, not be identified. There is no need to test blood coagulation; fine needle puncture is also safe in the case of coagulopathy.

Gall bladder puncture can safely be performed with the ultrasound-guided fine needle technique.[21,22] There is no need to approach the gall bladder transhepatically; any approach is safe. The gall bladder and large bile ducts should never be damaged with a wide core needle, which may lead to rupture, vagal reactions and shock. These drawbacks do not apply to fine needle puncture, which is a safe technique. Puncture of the gall bladder should be avoided in the case of extrahepatic bile duct obstruction, where there is a chance of inducing rupture or bile leakage. Sampling of bile for cytology and culture is especially important in cats, in which cholangitis is one of the most frequent hepatobiliary disorders.

FORCEPS BIOPSY DURING LAPAROSCOPY

The liver may be approached by laparoscopy.[23] This procedure makes it possible to identify local changes if they are visible at the liver surface. Samples may also be obtained in a directed manner from lesional sites. The usual way to obtain tissue during laparoscopy is with a forceps. The tissue comes from the subcapsular superficial region, which may not be representative. Subcapsular fibrosis may be normal and these superficial samples may give a misleading non-representative impression. Furthermore, forceps biopsies are often prone to compression artifacts.[3,4] It is also possible to obtain deeper True-cut needle samples through an endoscope, which may give a better representation. The advantage of possible directed sampling of local abnormalities has become obsolete as a result of the availability of ultrasonography and ultrasound-guided needle biopsy. Laparoscopy is time-consuming and requires general anesthesia, which are distinct disadvantages compared with the True-cut or Menghini technique.

SURGICAL WEDGE BIOPSY

Surgical biopsies may provide larger samples than needle or forceps biopsies. In order to avoid non-representative subcapsular fibrosis it is important to take wedge samples at least at 1 cm, preferably 2 cm deep. In human liver pathology, multiple deep needle biopsies are considered to be superior over wedge biopsies, which are necessarily always more superficial. Only in the case of visible superficial lesions are wedge samples held to be superior.[4] If wedge biopsies are sampled from diffusely affected livers, it is advisable to take two samples in order to ensure that representation is as good as possible. Obviously, visible local changes can be sampled during surgery. Although wedge samples are large, this is insufficient reason to perform abdominal surgery simply to obtain liver tissue. Surgery is too crude a tool, bearing in mind the invasiveness, unnecessary anesthetic risk and expense. Wide-core needle samples are adequate and are minimally invasive in comparison with surgery.

DIAGNOSTIC ACCURACY OF LIVER TISSUE SAMPLING

Liver histopathology is a cornerstone of the process in the diagnosis and evaluation of liver diseases. Sampling of liver tissue is too often omitted by clinicians, with the result that their conclusions are not based on solid evidence. The thresholds for taking biopsies should therefore be as low as possible. The considerations discussed in this chapter may help towards the development of a confident approach for adequate sampling (for a summary,

Table 2.1 Summary of advantages, disadvantages and requirements of different liver biopsy techniques

	True-cut	True-cut gun	Menghini	Fine needle	Laparoscopic forceps or needle	Surgical wedge
Local anesthesia	+	+	+	−		
General anesthesia					+	+
2–3 samples required	+	+	+	−	+	+
Histology and cytology	+	+	+	−	+	+
Only cytology	−	−	−	+	−	−
Ultrasound guided	+	+	−			
Blind technique	−	−	+	+/−	−	−
Invasiveness	+	+	+	+/−	++	+++
Suitable for cats[a]	+	−[b]	-	+	+	+
Suitable for dogs	+	+	+	+	+	+
Experience required	−	+/−	+	−	+	−
Cost	+	+[c]	−	−	++	+++

[a] For cats general anesthesia is advised; [b] not for use in cats, which may develop severe, even lethal vagotonic reactions; [c] less expensive in large clinics.

see Table 2.1). A tissue biopsy sample is only a small part of the entire organ and therefore, it may not be adequately representative. However, there are considerations that can be taken into account in getting as close to the truth as possible. In human medicine, specialists in liver pathology have developed criteria,[3,4] which according to the veterinary pathologists who have contributed to this book, are also relevant for veterinary medicine. First, at least two good samples should be examined, but if possible, three such samples are preferred. This recommendation goes for every technique in use for liver tissue sampling. Each individual needle biopsy sample should have a minimal core length of 1 cm, but 2 cm is much better. If possible, three such samples are preferred. The advantage of needle biopsies is that they gather tissue from as deep as 3 cm, or if obtained with ultrasound guidance, from any depth. Adequate sampling depth improves the representation of the entire liver considerably. The diameter of the needle, either True-cut or Menghini, is also important for obtaining adequate representation. The recommendation is that 14 G needles are used for medium and large sized dogs, and 16 G needles for smaller dogs and cats. Local lesions should not only be sampled in the center, but also in the periphery

of the process. This is especially important in cases of malignancy.

True-cut and Menghini biopsies, when performed with understanding, are adequately representative and provide enough tissue for any form of histopathological examination. A final remark is that the clinician may find it hard to obtain enough tissue in certain cases; however, it is always worthwhile to submit a sample, even if it is not optimal. If crucial changes happen to be present in a small sample, this may still lead to a confident diagnosis.

RECOMMENDED STAINING TECHNIQUES FOR PATHOLOGISTS

In general, experienced pathologists tend to use only a limited number of stains to assess liver tissues. Additional techniques may only be necessary for very specific questions. The most useful staining methods are summarized here:

- The routine stain for all samples is hematoxylin and eosin (H&E). For many cases this stain alone is adequate for good evaluation of the tissue.
- Collapse due to necrosis, fibrosis, or architectural changes such as cirrhosis can best be eval-

uated with the reticulin stain according to Gordon and Sweet, Sirius red, Masson's trichrome stain, or Van Gieson's stain.

Additional stains may be used to detect or confirm specific substances such as glycogen (periodic acid Schiff (PAS) stain), ceroid-lipofuscine (prolonged Ziehl-Neelsen and diastase-PAS stain),

copper (rubeanic acid or Rhodanine stain), iron (Perl's stain), amyloid (Congo red or Stokes stain), or bilirubin (Fouchet's stain).

There are many immunohistochemical staining methods that can often be performed on formalin-fixed and paraffin embedded tissue slices. However, these stains often work better in unfixed frozen tissue.

References

1. Szatmari V, Rothuizen J, van den Ingh TS, et al. Ultrasonographic findings in dogs with hyperammonemia: 90 cases (2000–2002). J Am Vet Med Assoc 2004;224(5):717–727.
2. Szatmari V. Ultrasonography of portosystemic shunting in dogs. Doppler studies before, during and after surgery. Thesis, Utrecht University. December 2004.
3. Desmet V, Fevery J. Liver biopsy. In: Hayes PC, ed. Investigations in hepatology. Baillière's clinical gastroenterology, vol. 9, no. 4. London: Baillière Tindall; 1995:811–828.
4. Geller SA. Liver biopsy for the nonpathologist. In: Gitnick G, ed. Principles and practice of gastroenterology and hepatology. 2nd edn. Norwalk: Appleton and Lange; 1994:1023–1036.
5. Badylak SF, Dodds WJ, Van Vleet JF. Plasma coagulation factor abnormalities in dogs with naturally occurring hepatic disease. Am J Vet Res 1983;44(12):2336–2340.
6. Badylak SF, Van Vleet JF. Alterations of prothrombin time and activated partial thromboplastin time in dogs with hepatic disease. Am J Vet Res 1981;42(12):2053–2056.
7. Bigge LA, Brown DJ, Penninck DG. Correlation between coagulation profile findings and bleeding complications after ultrasound-guided biopsies: 434 cases (1993–1996). J Am Anim Hosp Assoc 2001;37(3):228–233.
8. Mount ME, Kim BU, Kass PH. Use of a test for proteins induced by vitamin K absence or antagonism in diagnosis of anticoagulant poisoning in dogs: 325 cases (1987–1997). J Am Vet Med Assoc 2003;222(2):194–198.
9. Webster CRL. History, clinical signs, and physical findings in hepatobiliary disease. In: Ettinger SJ, Feldman EC, eds. Textbook of veterinary internal medicine. St. Louis: Elsevier Saunders; 2005:1422–1434.
10. Lisciandro SC, Hohenhaus A, Brooks M. Coagulation abnormalities in 22 cats with naturally occurring liver disease. J Vet Intern Med 1998;12(2):71–75.
11. Center SA, Warner K, Corbett J, et al. Proteins invoked by vitamin K absence and clotting times in clinically ill cats. J Vet Intern Med 2000;14(3):292–297.
12. Rothuizen J. Diseases of the liver and biliary tract. In: Dunn J, ed. Textbook of small animal medicine. London: Saunders; 1999:448–497.
13. Feldman EC, Ettinger SJ. Percutaneous transthoracic liver biopsy in the dog. J Am Vet Med Assoc 1976;169(8):805–810.
14. Bunch S. Diagnostic tests for the hepatobiliary system. In: Nelson RW, Couto CG, eds. Small animal internal medicine. St. Louis: Mosby; 2003:483–505.
15. Niza MM, Ferreira AJ, Peleteiro MC, et al. Bacteriological study of the liver in dogs. J Small Anim Pract 2004;45(8):401–404.
16. Cole TL, Center SA, Flood SN, et al. Diagnostic comparison of needle and wedge biopsy specimens of the liver in dogs and cats. J Am Vet Med Assoc 2002;220(10):1483–1490.
17. de Rycke LM, van Bree HJ, Simoens PJ. Ultrasound-guided tissue-core biopsy of liver, spleen and kidney in normal dogs. Vet Radiol Ultrasound 1999;40(3):294–299.
18. Simpson JW, Else RW. Diagnostic value of tissue biopsy in gastrointestinal and liver disease. Vet Rec 1987;120(10):230-233.
19. Stockhaus C, Van Den Ingh T, Rothuizen J, et al. A multistep approach in the cytologic evaluation of liver biopsy samples of dogs with hepatic diseases. Vet Pathol 2004;41(5):461–470.
20. Weiss DJ, Moritz A. Liver cytology. Vet Clin North Am Small Anim Pract 2002;32(6):1267–1291.
21. Rivers BJ, Walter PA, Johnston GR, et al. Acalculous cholecystitis in four canine cases: ultrasonographic findings and use of ultrasonographic-guided, percutaneous cholecystocentesis in diagnosis. J Am Anim Hosp Assoc 1997;33(3):207–214.
22. Savary-Bataille KC, Bunch SE, Spaulding KA, et al. Percutaneous ultrasound-guided cholecystocentesis in healthy cats. J Vet Intern Med 2003;17(3):298–303.
23. Richter KP. Laparoscopy in dogs and cats. Vet Clin North Am Small Anim Pract 2001;31(4):707–727.

Chapter **3**

Ultrasonographic identification and characterization of congenital portosystemic shunts and portal hypertensive disorders in dogs and cats

Viktor Szatmári, Jan Rothuizen

CHAPTER CONTENTS

INTRODUCTION

In the first part of this chapter the hemodynamic, anatomical and pathophysiological features of canine portal vein disorders are described. Understanding these principles is necessary for correct interpretation of the ultrasonographic images. In the second part of the chapter an ultrasonographic scanning protocol is described, which is recommended for use in the thorough evaluation of the portal venous system. A short section at the end discusses the specific features of feline portal vein disorders.

NORMAL ABDOMINAL VASCULAR ANATOMY IN DOGS

The aorta, the caudal vena cava (CVC) and the portal vein (PV) are the three great abdominal vessels, which all run parallel to the vertebral column. The aorta is the most dorsal and its major branches from cranial to caudal are: the celiac, the cranial mesenteric, the right and left renal arteries, and before the final trifurcation, the right and left external iliac arteries.[1] The celiac artery branches further into three arteries, of which the largest is the common hepatic artery, which runs cranially between the PV and the CVC (Fig. 3.1). All the above vessels can be visualized with ultrasound.

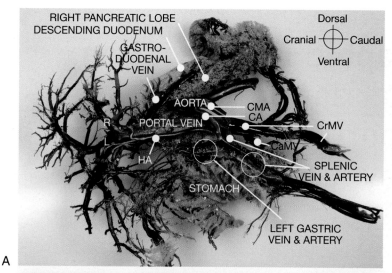

A

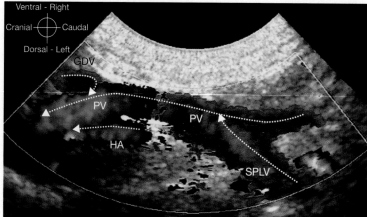

B

Figure 3.1 Normal canine abdominal blood vessels.
(A) Corrosion cast of the portal vein (blue) and the cranial part of the abdominal aorta (red) in an adult normal beagle. Before preparation the spleen, jejunum, ileum and colon were removed and the descending duodenum was retracted. R – right portal branch; L – left portal branch; CA – celiac artery; CMA – cranial mesenteric artery; HA – hepatic artery; CrMV – cranial mesenteric vein, CaMV – caudal mesenteric vein.
(B) Color Doppler ultrasound image of a normal portal vein (PV) of a Yorkshire terrier. The diameter of the portal vein is uniform along its whole length. The image was made via the right flank with the dog in left lateral recumbency (plane 4). Dotted arrows indicate the direction of blood flow. GDV – gastroduodenal vein; SPLV – splenic vein; HA – hepatic artery. (Reproduced from Szatmári V et al. Standard planes for ultrasonographic examination of the portal system in dogs. J Am Vet Med Assoc 2004; 224:713–716, with permission.)

The smallest intrahepatic branches of the hepatic artery terminate in the hepatic sinusoids.

The CVC is formed by the confluence of the right and left common iliac veins at the level of the aortic trifurcation. The CVC runs ventral to the aorta and after entering the thoracic cavity it terminates in the right atrium. The abdominal CVC collects the blood of the left and the right renal veins, and as it passes through the liver it collects the blood of the hepatic veins. The hepatic veins drain the blood of the hepatic sinusoids and are straight vessels running through the liver lobes in a craniomedial direction. The left gonadal vein (ovarian vein in females and testicular vein in males) enters the left renal vein, whereas the right gonadal vein is a direct tributary of the caudal vena cava.[2] The renal and hepatic veins can be visualized with ultrasound, but the gonadal veins cannot be seen because of their small diameter.

The PV is formed by the confluence of the cranial and caudal mesenteric veins.[2] The PV collects the blood of the splenic vein at the level where the celiac artery originates from the aorta, as well as the blood of the gastroduodenal vein immediately caudal to the portal bifurcation. The left gastric vein is a tributary of the splenic vein. The right gastric vein is either a tributary of the gastroduodenal vein or of the PV. In the latter case it enters the PV directly cranial to the gastroduodenal vein after running along the lesser curvature of the stomach.[3] At the hilus of the liver the trunk of the PV bifurcates into a larger left and a smaller right portal branch. The right branch courses dorsally, the left one ventrally. The right branch supplies the right lateral and the caudate hepatic lobes, whereas the left branch supplies the left lateral, left medial, quadrate and right medial lobes. The smallest portal branches terminate in the hepatic sinusoids where their blood mixes with the hepatic arterial blood. The splenic vein, the gastroduodenal vein and the left and right portal branches can be visualized with ultrasound.

The right azygos vein is a thin vessel that runs dorsal to the aorta and after passing through the diaphragm it enters the cranial vena cava, which later terminates in the right atrium.[2]

The CVC and the azygos veins, together with their tributaries, belong to the systemic venous system, and the PV, together with its tributaries, form the portal venous system. No macroscopic communication exists between the systemic and the portal veinous systems.

Portosystemic shunting occurs when anomalous veins allow the portal blood to enter the systemic veins directly without first flowing through the hepatic sinusoids.[4] Portosystemic shunting can occur via acquired portosystemic collaterals or via congenital portosystemic shunts.[4–6]

DIAGNOSTIC APPROACH TO DOGS SUSPECTED OF HAVING PORTOSYSTEMIC SHUNTING

Because portosystemic shunting can cause a great variety of clinical signs, and ultrasonographic visualization of the anomalous veins has been a diagnostic challenge, measuring fasting venous blood ammonia level has become a routine procedure to justify or rule out the presence of portosystemic shunting.[7,8]

Determining the blood ammonia level before performing an abdominal ultrasound examination can greatly increase the positive and negative predictive values of ultrasonography in finding the anomalous vein since chronic hyperammonemia can only be caused by a few diseases such as congenital portosystemic shunts (CPSSs), acquired portosystemic collaterals (APSCs), or urea cycle enzyme deficiency.[9,10] Differentiating these conditions non-invasively (e.g. by ultrasound) is crucial because CPSSs is the only disease that requires sur-

gical treatment; the other two do not. Some other diseases may also cause hyperammonemia, but they can be differentiated from the above-mentioned disorders by clinical examination and laboratory tests.[9]

Abdominal ultrasonography can readily diagnose CPSSs in non-sedated dogs. Moreover, the anatomy of the shunting vessel (i.e. intra- or extrahepatic) can be precisely determined.[9,11–13] This knowledge is important not only for the surgeon, but also for predicting the prognosis.[14] The other great advantage of ultrasonography is that the other conditions causing elevated blood ammonia and bile acids levels, such as APSCs, may also be diagnosed.[9]

PATHOPHYSIOLOGY OF CANINE PORTAL HYPERTENSION

APSCs are formed as the result of sustained intrahepatic or prehepatic portal hypertension by enlargement of extrahepatic rudimentary vessels, through which no blood normally passes.[5,6] The term 'prehepatic' refers to disorders that affect the portal vein (i.e. extravascular compression or intravascular obstruction).[6] The term 'intrahepatic' refers to the diseases of the liver itself, and the term 'posthepatic' refers to conditions that affect the thoracic CVC or the heart.[6] Posthepatic portal hypertension (e.g. right-sided congestive heart failure) never results in APSC-formation because not only the portal, but also the caval pressure increases.[6] Posthepatic portal hypertension results in an enlarged liver and dilated hepatic veins due to congestion, whereas prehepatic portal hypertension results in a small liver due to insufficient portal venous perfusion. In intrahepatic portal hypertension the small or normal-sized liver has a slightly or severely abnormal (echo-)structure. A common, but not consistently occurring consequence of any kind of portal hypertension is the accumulation of free abdominal fluid (pure or modified transudate).[6]

Acquired portosystemic collaterals in dogs

Collateral-formation is a compensatory mechanism to maintain normal portal pressure by allowing the portal blood to be drained into the lower pressure systemic veins.[5,6] Collateral veins run simultane-

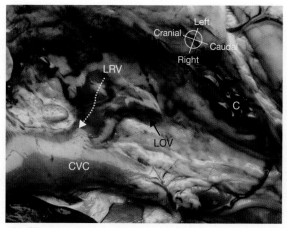 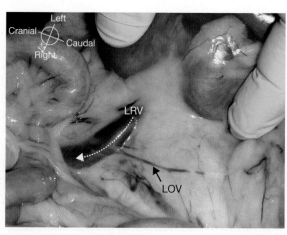

A   B

Figure 3.2 The left gonadal vein, which is a normal tributary of the left renal vein.
(A) Dilated left ovarian vein (LOV) in a 5-month-old female great Dane with spleno-renal collaterals as a result of sustained portal hypertension of hepatic origin. C – conglomeration of collateral vessels; CVC – caudal vena cava; LRV – left renal vein.
(B) Normal left ovarian vein in a 9-month-old female Labrador retriever. The left ovarian vein (LOV) enters the left renal vein from the caudal aspect. It is much thinner than the left renal vein (LRV).

ously in several anatomical ways, however dogs tend to consistently develop the so called spleno-renal (actually splenic-left gonadal vein) collaterals.[5,6] As a result of the spleno-renal collateral circulation the left gonadal vein (testicular vein in males and ovarian vein in females) becomes dilated[15] because a portion of the portal venous blood is forced to flow via the splenic vein through the preexisting embryonic connections to the left gonadal vein, and from here through the left renal vein eventually to the CVC (Fig. 3.2).

In addition to the dilated left gonadal vein, the origin of an APSC can occasionally be found with ultrasound at the point where congenital extra-hepatic spleno-caval shunts arise from the PV (see later in this chapter). In these cases, normal flow may be seen in the PV caudal to the APSC-origin and hepatofugal (i.e. away from the liver) flow cranial to it (Fig. 3.3A). In other dogs with portal hypertension the flow in the PV may be so slow that no color signals can be detected (Fig. 3.3B).

Etiology of canine portal hypertension

Once the presence of portal hypertension has been established, e.g. by visualizing a dilated left gonadal vein, the next diagnostic step is to identify the underlying cause. Ultrasonography is able to determine the cause of prehepatic portal hypertension as well as diagnose arterioportal fistula. Intrahepatic portal hypertension may only be suspected with ultrasound.

Prehepatic portal hypertension can be caused by compression of the portal vein by a neoplasia or a cyst or by an obstruction of the portal vein by a thrombus or a tumor. Both conditions can readily be diagnosed with ultrasound.

Congenital arterioportal fistula is a developmental anomaly characterized by a direct connection between a portal venous and a hepatic arterial branch.[9,16] The high arterial pressure is responsible for the classical ultrasonographic changes:

1. Extremely dilated and tortuous portal branch in a liver lobe
2. Hepatofugal flow in the PV (with a variable or an arterial Doppler spectrum
3. APSCs (Fig. 3.4).[9]

Ascites (pure transudate) is usually present.

Intrahepatic portal hypertension must be suspected in dogs with a high blood ammonia level if ultrasonography discloses a dilated left gonadal vein and excludes arterioportal fistula and compression or obstruction of the PV. Intrahepatic

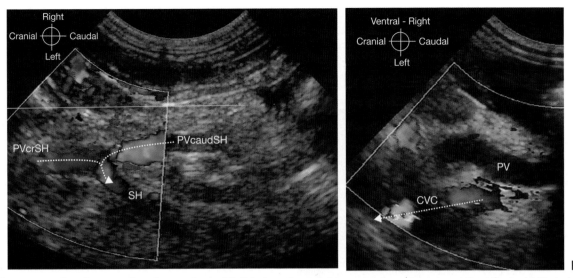

Figure 3.3 Portal venous flow in two dogs with intrahepatic portal hypertension. (Reproduced from Szatmári V et al. Ultrasonographic findings in dogs with hyperammonemia: 90 cases (2000–2002). J Am Vet Med Assoc 2004; 224:717–727, with permission.)
(A) Color Doppler ultrasound image of the portal vein and the origin of an acquired portosystemic collateral (SH) in a 5-year-old West Highland white terrier with sustained portal hypertension of hepatic origin. Cranial to the collateral-origin (PVcrSH) hepatofugal portal flow can be seen. Note that the anomalous vein (SH) runs caudally. Dotted arrows indicate the direction of blood flow. In the portal vein caudal to the collateral origin (PVcaudSH) normal flow can be seen.
(B) Color Doppler ultrasound image of the portal vein in a 6.5-year-old female Jack Russell terrier with sustained portal hypertension due to primary hypoplasia of the portal vein shows undetectably slow flow in the portal vein. Note that no color signals are seen in the portal vein (PV), whereas aliasing artefact is apparent in the caudal vena cava (CVC). The dotted arrow indicates the direction of blood flow.

portal hypertension can be caused by parenchymal liver diseases (chronic hepatitis of various etiologies)[17–19] or anomalies of the portal branches [e.g. primary hypoplasia of the portal vein (PHPV)].[9,20] Diagnosis and differentiation between these conditions require histopathologic examination of liver biopsy specimens.

In mild cases of PHPV, portal hypertension does not develop, hence blood ammonia level remains low, however in severe cases, APSCs develop as a consequence of sustained pre- and intrahepatic portal hypertension.[9,20]

Primary hypoplasia of the portal vein is simultaneously present with arterioportal fistula and might accompany CPSSs.[9] When a CPSS and PHPV coincide in a dog, PHPV cannot be diagnosed preoperatively. In these dogs, portal hypertension and APSCs will not develop because there is an already existing connection between the portal and the systemic veins (i.e. the CPSS).[21] Currently, the earliest time point when PHPV can be suspected in a dog with CPSS is during surgical attenuation of extrahepatic CPSSs, with intraoperative Doppler ultrasonography.[22]

CONGENITAL PORTOSYSTEMIC SHUNTS IN DOGS

Portosystemic shunting is considered to be congenital when a single, usually large-bore vein is present without a concurrent portal hypertension.[4] Congenital portosystemic shunts are classified as intrahepatic and extrahepatic. Since a CPSS has an equal or larger diameter compared to the PV-segment caudal to the shunt, it offers a lower resistance path for the blood to reach the systemic veins than through the hepatic sinusoids. As blood tends to flow towards the lowest possible resistance, the vast majority of the portal blood flows via the shunt because hepatic sinusoids represent much higher resistance to flow. Therefore, the liver receives no or only a small fraction of the portal blood, which is insufficient for normal hepatic development and function.[4,23]

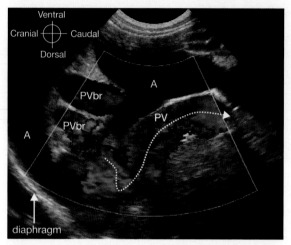

Figure 3.4 Congenital arterio-portal fistula. Color Doppler ultrasound image of the liver of a 6-month-old male American Staffordshire terrier reveals dilated portal branches (PVbr) in the affected liver lobe. The flow direction in the portal vein (PV) is hepatofugal indicated by the dotted arrow. A – ascites. (Reproduced from Szatmári V et al. Ultrasonographic findings in dogs with hyperammonemia: 90 cases (2000–2002). J Am Vet Med Assoc 2004; 224:717–727, with permission.)

Intrahepatic congenital porto-caval shunts

Intrahepatic porto-caval shunts occur predominantly in large breed dogs,[24] particularly in Bernese mountain dogs and retrievers. Intrahepatic CPSSs originate either from the left or from the right portal branch and appear as the direct continuations of the PV, as the diameters of the shunt and of the affected portal branch are the same as that of the PV.[9] Because the majority of blood flows through the portal branch that continues as the shunt, the contralateral portal branch remains very thin due to hypoperfusion. All intrahepatic CPSSs terminate in the CVC either directly or via a hepatic vein.[25] The intrahepatic CPSS is usually a single vein, but exceptionally they can have two loops.[9,26]

Intrahepatic CPSSs that originate from the left portal branch run cranioventrally and to the left (similar to a normal left portal branch) to the diaphragm, then turn abruptly dorsally to enter the CVC via a dilated segment of the left hepatic vein.[25] In these dogs the right portal branch is very thin (Fig. 3.5).[9]

Intrahepatic CPSSs that originate from the right portal branch appear as the direct continuation of the right portal branch (Fig. 3.6). The dilated right portal branch runs consistently dorsolaterally and to the right from the PV, like a normal right portal branch, but then, instead of tapering, it turns medi-

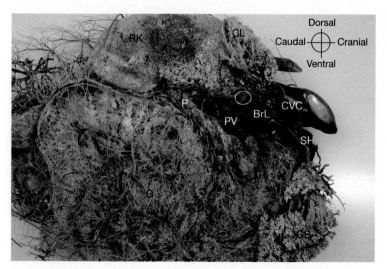

Figure 3.5 Patent ductus venosus. Corrosion cast of a left divisional intrahepatic portocaval shunt of a 2-month-old Irish wolfhound. The portal vein (PV) has the same diameter as the left portal branch (BrL) and the shunt (SH). The right portal branch (○ blue) is very narrow, however the corresponding hepatic arterial branch (○ red) is relatively wide. CVC – caudal vena cava; RK - right kidney; AO – aorta; CL – caudate liver lobe; P – pancreas; G – guts; GB – gallbladder.

Figure 3.6 Congenital intrahepatic portocaval shunt from the right portal branch. Corrosion cast of a central divisional intrahepatic portocaval shunt of a 7-month-old mixed breed dog 3 months after partial shunt ligation. The portal vein (PV) continues via the right portal branch (arrow) to the caudal vena cava (CVC). Three months after shunt attenuation the left portal branch (BrL) is still rather narrow. There is ligature around the shunt. The PV and CVC slightly caudal to the liver have been removed. HV – hepatic vein.

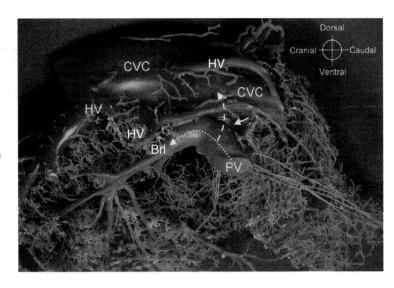

ally to enter the CVC.[9,25] The dorsolaterally running segment is either short or long (i.e. central and right divisional shunt, respectively). Whatever morphology a right-sided intrahepatic CPSS has, the left portal branch is severely underdeveloped.

A dog with simultaneous intrahepatic CPSS and arterioportal fistula has been reported.[27]

Extrahepatic congenital portosystemic shunts

Extrahepatic portosystemic shunts occur mostly in small breeds, particularly in Maltese dogs, miniature schnauzers and small terriers (Yorkshire, Jack Russell, cairn), but are occasionally seen in large breeds. Extrahepatic CPSSs originate from the splenic vein, from the right gastric vein, or from both as communicating loops, and enter either the abdominal CVC or the thorax: the spleno-caval and right gastric-caval enter the abdominal caudal vena cava, the spleno-azygos and right gastric-azygos enter the thorax.[9] Shunts with two loops (one arising from the right gastric vein and the other one from the splenic vein) are categorized as right gastric shunts because the right gastric vein is the main loop and this has an identical morphology with the single shunts that arise from the right gastric vein. Though extrahepatic CPSSs are named after a portal tributary, they all divert the blood of the PV via a short and dilated segment of the involved tributary. Extrahepatic CPSSs with anatomy other than the four types described above, are extremely rare in dogs.[28]

Extrahepatic CPSSs arising from the splenic vein

Spleno-caval shunts are the most common type of congenital extrahepatic CPSSs. They usually form a short loop between the PV and the CVC. Although the anomalous vein may have a long cranially extending loop, the points of origin and termination are always the same. As the point of shunt origin is very close to the point where the splenic vein enters the PV and the short segment of the splenic vein that is between the PV and the shunt origin is dilated and the flow hepatofugal (i.e. away from the liver) in it, the CPSS seems to originate from the PV itself and the splenic vein seems to enter the shunting vessel (Fig. 3.7). The origin of the spleno-caval shunts is slightly cranial to the level where the celiac artery originates from the aorta (i.e. approximately at the level of the cranial pole of the right kidney, Fig. 3.7B). The termination of the spleno-caval shunts in the CVC is always at the same point, i.e. slightly cranial to the level of the shunt-origin (Fig 3.8A).[9,13]

In cases of spleno-azygos shunts, the shunting vessel approaches the CVC at the point where the spleno-caval shunts terminate, but instead of

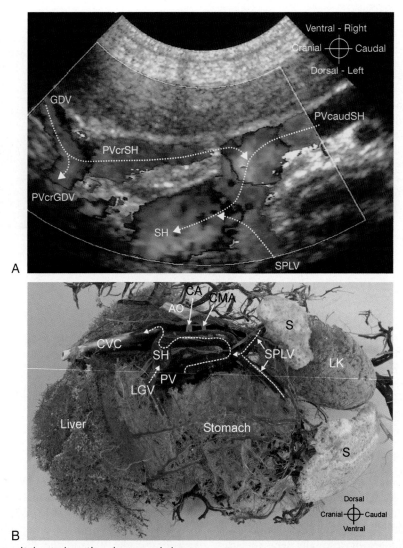

Figure 3.7 Congenital extrahepatic spleno-caval shunt.

(A) Color Doppler ultrasound image of the portal vein in longitudinal section made via the right flank with the dog in left lateral recumbency (plane 4). The shunt (SH) originates from the splenic vein (SPLV), very close to the point where the SPLV normally enters the portal vein. Both the intestinal and the splenic blood are diverted. In the portal vein segment between the shunt origin and the entering point of the gastroduodenal vein (PVcrSH) the flow is hepatofugal. This PVcrSH is thinner than the portal vein caudal to the shunt origin (PVcaudSH). Cranial to the entering point of the gastroduodenal vein (GDV) the portal flow is hepatopetal (PVcrGDV). Dotted arrows indicate the direction of blood flow. (Reproduced from Szatmári V et al. Ultrasonographic evaluation of partially attenuated congenital extrahepatic portosystemic shunts in 14 dogs. Vet Rec 2004; 155:448–456, with permission.)

(B) Corrosion cast of the abdominal blood vessels of a 2-month-old cairn terrier. The veins are blue and the arteries are red. The shunt (SH) terminates in the caudal vena cava (CVC) slightly cranial to the point where the celiac artery (CA) originates from the aorta (AO). The left gastric vein (LGV) and both the dorsal and ventral branches of the splenic vein (SPLV) enter the SH. The portal vein (PV) is thin cranial to the SH origin. Dotted arrows indicate the direction of blood flow in a living animal. CMA – cranial mesenteric artery; LK – left kidney; S – spleen (the middle part of the spleen has been removed).

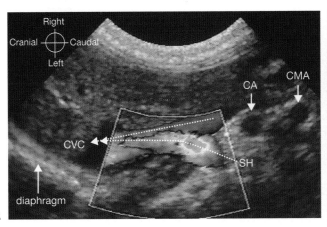

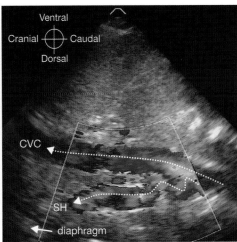

Figure 3.8   Congenital extrahepatic portosystemic shunts in two dogs. Color Doppler ultrasound images show the termination of congenital extrahepatic portosystemic shunts. The transducer was positioned caudal to the last right rib (flank) with the dog in dorsal recumbency. Dotted arrows indicate the direction of blood flow. (Reproduced from Szatmári V et al. Ultrasonographic findings in dogs with hyperammonemia: 90 cases (2000–2002). J Am Vet Med Assoc 2004; 224:717–727, with permission.)

(A) Spleno-caval shunt in a 3-month-old female cairn terrier at the point where the shunt (SH) enters the caudal vena cava (CVC). This point is always located slightly cranial to the point where the celiac artery (CA) originates from the aorta. CMA – cranial mesenteric artery.

(B) Spleno-azygos shunt in a 3.5-month-old male Jack Russell terrier. The shunting vessel (SH) runs dorsal to the CVC, and enters the thorax.

entering it the shunting vessel runs dorsal to the CVC and eventually enters the thorax (Fig. 3.8B). The point of origin of these spleno-azygos shunts is the same as that of the spleno-caval shunts (Fig 3.7A).

Since the diameter of the shunt is always wider than that of the PV caudal to the shunt origin the PV cranial to the shunt origin and the intrahepatic portal branches remain hypoperfused. Therefore, the PV segment cranial to the shunt origin is always thinner than the PV segment caudal to the shunt origin. In most cases of extrahepatic CPSSs the left and right portal branches are also very thin. When they have a relatively normal diameter, color Doppler shows an undetectably slow or very slow hepatopetal (i.e. towards the liver) flow in them. The flow-direction in the PV segment cranial to the shunt origin is hepatofugal in most dogs, however it could be slow hepatopetal (i.e. flow to the liver) or alternating ('to-and-fro'). The blood of the gastroduodenal vein was found to be responsible for the hepatofugal flow because the gastroduodenal blood finds lower resistance to flow towards the

shunt (i.e. to caudal) than towards the hepatic sinusoids (Fig. 3.7A).

The morphology of the APSCs that originate from the PV can be very similar to that of congenital extrahepatic spleno-caval shunts (Figs 3.3A, 3.7A). Moreover, in both cases hepatofugal portal flow cranial to the origin of the anomalous vein could be seen. The differences are: an APSC runs caudally from its origin and tends to disappear among the intestines; furthermore the diameters of the PV cranial and caudal to the APSC origin are roughly equal (Fig. 3.3A). In contrast, congenital extrahepatic spleno-caval or spleno-azygos shunts tend to run cranially from the origin and can always be followed to their terminations (CVC or diaphragm). Thirdly, the PV segment that is cranial to the origin of a spleno-caval or a spleno-azygos shunt is always thinner than the PV segment caudal to it (Fig. 3.7). Moreover, an APSC is thinner than the PV caudal to the anomalous vein, unlike in cases of CPSSs. The simultaneous presence of the dilated left gonadal vein proves that an extrahep-

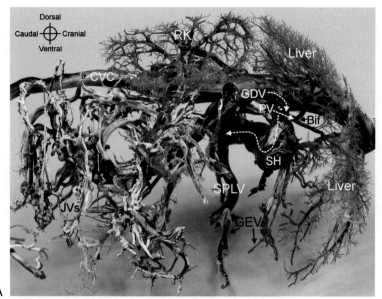

A

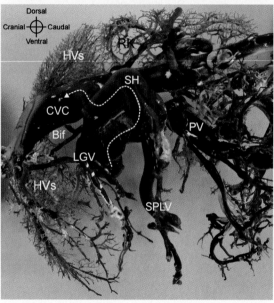

B

Figure 3.9 Right gastric-caval shunt with one shunt loop. Corrosion cast of the abdominal veins of a Dachshund with congenital extrahepatic right gastric-caval shunt. In this patient only the cranial shunt loop (SH) has developed. The left kidney has been removed. RK – right kidney.
(A) The shunt (SH) originates at the point where the gastroduodenal vein (GDV) enters the portal vein (PV). The right gastric vein is a tributary of the GDV. The PV caudal to the SH origin is thinner than the SH and becomes very thin cranial to the SH origin. The right portal branch runs to the dorsal aspect and the left portal branch to the ventral aspect. Bif – portal bifurcation; CVC – caudal vena cava; GEV – left and right gastroepiploic veins; JVs – jejunal veins; SPLV – splenic vein.
(B) The portal vein (PV) becomes very thin cranial to the origin of the SH. Compare the PV diameter caudal to the SH with that just caudal to the PV bifurcation (Bif). Both the splenic vein (SPLV) and the left gastric vein (LGV) enter the SH. The SH terminates in the caudal vena cava (CVC). HVs – hepatic veins.

atic anomalous vein originating from the PV with a hepatofugal flow is the origin of an APSC and not that of a CPSS.[9]

Extrahepatic CPSSs arising from the right gastric vein

Right gastric-caval shunts have either one or two loops. In the former case only the cranial loop (right gastric-caval loop) is present (Fig. 3.9). In the latter case both the cranial loop and the caudal loop (spleno-caval loop) are present and they anastomose before entering the CVC (Fig. 3.10). The cranial loop arises from the right gastric vein and the morphology of this loop varies slightly depending on whether the right gastric vein is a tributary of the gastroduodenal vein or of the PV itself originating between the portal bifurcation and the gas-

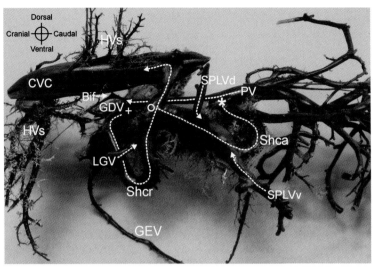

Figure 3.10 Right gastric–caval shunt with two shunt loops. Corrosion cast of the abdominal veins of a Yorkshire terrier with a right gastric–caval shunt. Both the cranial shunt loop (Shcr) and the caudal shunt loop (SHca) are present and they anastomose with each other (o). The portal vein (PV) becomes narrower cranial to the point of the Shca origin (*), and even more narrow cranial to the point of the Shcr origin (+). The Shcr originates at the point where the gastroduodenal vein (GDV) enters the PV. By surgical closure of the common trunk of the SH adjacent to the caudal vena cava (CVC) both shunt loops can be terminated. The arrows indicate the flow directions in the vessels in a living animal. Bif – portal bifurcation with the very thin right and left portal branches; HVs – hepatic veins; GEV – right and left gastroepiploic veins; SPLVv – ventral branch of the splenic vein; SPLVd – dorsal branch of the splenic vein. (The CVC has been removed caudal to the SH termination.)

troduodenal vein.[3] In both cases the shunt originates immediately caudal to the portal bifurcation via the dilated right gastric vein. When the right gastric vein is a direct tributary of the PV, the blood of the PV is drained via the dilated right gastric vein to the CVC. When the right gastric vein is a tributary of the gastroduodenal vein, the blood of the PV is drained via a short and dilated segment of the gastroduodenal vein through the right gastric vein into the CVC, and the blood of the gastroduodenal vein flows through the shunt (i.e. the right gastric vein) without reaching the PV first. Regardless of the anatomical variation of the right gastric vein, the course of the shunt (i.e. the right gastric vein) is always the same, namely it makes a long loop from the liver hilus first laterally to the left body wall, then from here to caudomedially, to eventually enter the CVC at the point where the spleno-caval shunts terminate (i.e. slightly cranial to the celiac artery, Fig. 3.11). The caudal shunt loop of a right-gastric-caval shunt resembles a spleno-caval shunt.

Exceptionally, the shunting vessel does not enter the CVC, but runs dorsal to it and enters the thorax (right gastric-azygos shunts).

All CPSSs that arise from the right gastric vein are very wide, with a diameter comparable to that of the CVC. At surgical exploration the cranial loop of the right gastric-caval shunt is found to follow the lesser curvature of the stomach, similarly to a normal right gastric vein. The caudal shunt loop, which is not consistently present, originates at the region where spleno-caval shunts are expected, but unlike spleno-caval CPSSs, it runs from caudal to cranial and not from ventral to dorsal like the spleno-caval shunts. The caudal loop drains the blood of the PV via the dilated segment of the splenic vein to the common trunk (Fig. 3.10). The PV becomes slightly thinner cranial to the origin of the caudal shunt loop (i.e. cranial to the splenic vein) with hepatopetal flow direction. The PV cranial to the origin of the cranial shunt loop is so thin that it cannot be visualized by ultrasound.[9] Right

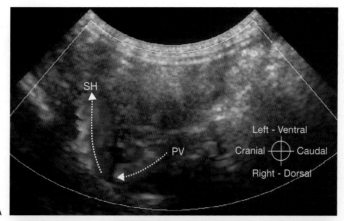

A

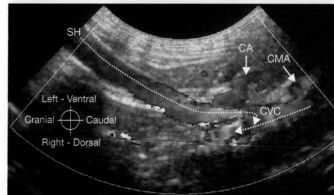

B

Figure 3.11   Right gastric-caval shunt. Color Doppler ultrasound images of (the cranial loop of) a congenital extrahepatic right gastric-caval shunt in a 6.5-month-old female Yorkshire terrier. The dog is in right lateral recumbency and the transducer is placed caudal to the last left rib (plane 6). Dotted arrows indicate the direction of flow.
(A) The shunt (SH) originates at the liver hilus and runs towards the left body wall making a roughly 90° angle with the portal vein (PV). The continuation of the shunt (traced caudally) is shown in (B). The PV cannot be seen cranial to the shunt origin because it is extremely thin due to hypoperfusion (see the corrosion cast).
(B) The shunt (SH) terminates in the caudal vena cava (CVC) cranial to the celiac artery (CA), similarly to a congenital extrahepatic spleno-caval shunt. Note the large caliber shunting vessel (SH) immediately under the left body wall. CMA – cranial mesenteric artery. (Reproduced from Szatmári V et al. Ultrasonographic findings in dogs with hyperammonemia: 90 cases (2000–2002). J Am Vet Med Assoc 2004; 224:717–727, with permission.)

gastric-caval shunts are frequently found in Maltese dogs.

HYPERAMMONEMIA WITHOUT PORTAL VEIN DISORDER

Urea cycle enzyme deficiency is a rare congenital metabolic disease.[10] Since no morphological changes are present, the abdominal ultrasound examination reveals normal-sized and structured liver and kidneys and the absence of vascular abnormalities.[9]

Peritoneal absorption of ammonia containing urine may result in hyperammonemia,[29] however this condition can easily be differentiated from portosystemic shunting by measuring high plasma creatinine concentration.

Irish wolfhound puppies have a physiological period of hyperammonemia.[30]

ABDOMINAL ULTRASONOGRAPHY OF PORTAL VEIN DISORDERS

Secondary changes

Before starting the examination of abdominal vessels, a detailed B-mode ultrasonographic study of the abdominal organs has to be performed. Determining the presence and amount of free abdominal fluid, the size and structure of the liver and kidneys is particularly important. The size of the left and right halves of the liver should be separately evaluated. The urinary bladder should also be examined for the presence of sediment or stone.

Typical findings in dogs with CPSS are a small liver, normal or enlarged kidneys (often with hyperechoic medulla) and no free abdominal fluid,[9,11,13] whereas dogs with APSCs have a small, normal-sized or asymmetrical liver (usually the left side is small and the right side is enlarged), a vari-

able amount of ascites (from none to a large amount) and slightly or markedly abnormal hepatic echo structure.[9] In acquired disease, the kidneys are of normal size, however they may be enlarged with congenital portal hypertensive disorders such as PHPV. A normal-sized liver and normalsized kidneys do not exclude CPSSs.

A large amount of free abdominal fluid may hinder ultrasonographic visualization of the abdominal vessels, but hyperammonemia in dogs with severe peritoneal effusion cannot possibly be the result of CPSSs or a urea cycle enzyme deficiency, since a dog with CPSS cannot have portal hypertension or hypoalbuminemia so severe that it would result in the formation of a large amount of transudate in the abdominal cavity.[6] A small amount of free abdominal fluid is normal in healthy puppies, hence it may also be seen in puppies with CPSSs or with urea cycle enzyme deficiency.[9]

The spleen is usually of normal size in dogs with both CPSSs and APSCs.[9] The reason why splenomegaly does not develop in dogs with portal hypertension could be that acquired spleno-renal collaterals are the most consistently developing APSCs in dogs, and these collateral veins prevent the spleen becoming congested.[9]

Diagnosis of CPSS is based on *visualizing* the anomalous vessel. Measuring portal flow velocities is of no use. It is recommended that ultrasonographic evaluation of the abdominal vasculature is performed in seven standard planes.[15]

Accurate recognition of CPSSs by ultrasound is only possible if the anomalous vein is traced from its origin to its termination, or the other way around. Finding the point where a CPSS enters the CVC may be easier than finding the origin of a CPSS,[13] however, finding a vein that enters the CVC does not mean that it is a CPSS because several other veins enter the CVC. In contrast, when a vein that originates from the PV displays hepatofugal flow, it is surely an extrahepatic CPSS or an APSC, even without knowing the point of its termination because in normal animals veins only enter and do not originate from the PV.

Diagnosing APSCs ultrasonographically requires a different approach from that of CPSSs because recognizably large collateral veins only occasionally arise directly from the PV, moreover they are thin and tortuous and are usually hidden among the intestines. Therefore, their origins and paths can only exceptionally be ultrasonographically revealed. However, the dilated left gonadal vein, i.e. the termination of the spleno-renal collaterals, has been found to be a highly specific and sensitive indicator of APSCs in dogs, and its ultrasonographic visualization is simple (Fig. 3.12).[9]

'**Double caudal vena cava**' refers to an innocent congenital anomaly: the left and right common iliac veins fuse to form the CVC in a more cranial position than usual, namely between the left and right renal veins.[31] Thus, the left renal vein enters the left common iliac vein and the right renal vein enters the CVC. The left and right common iliac veins have the same diameters and run symmetrically on the respective side of the aorta (Fig. 3.13). The only significance of this anomaly is that ultrasonographically the left common iliac vein may be mistaken for a dilated left gonadal vein.[9] However, careful examination can overcome this mistake. Of course, a 'double caudal vena cava' does not cause a high blood ammonia level, but it can be simultaneously present with a CPSS or with APSCs.

Machine settings

Color Doppler parameters should be adjusted with care so that a vessel is uniformly colored. Namely, the color gain must be set so that color signals are seen in the entire lumen of a given vessel, but not outside the vessel. Traditionally, flow towards the transducer is coded with red, and flow away from the transducer with blue. Higher flow velocities are coded with lighter hues of the appropriate color. The pulse repetition frequency (PRF or scale) should also be appropriately adjusted, since a given PRF setting is able to detect only a limited range of velocities.[32] If the PRF is set too high, slow flow may be missed. When the flow velocity is higher than the upper limit of the velocity range set that belongs to that particular PRF setting, then aliasing artefact occurs. Aliasing artefact means that if a flow velocity is higher than the upper limit of the velocity range belonging to a particular PRF, no more lighter shades are available of the appropriate color; therefore these velocities will be coded with the opposite color, i.e. the color that indicates flow to the opposite direction.[32]

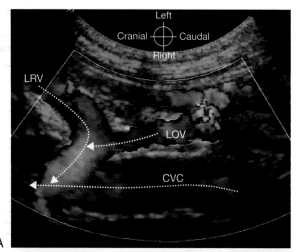

A

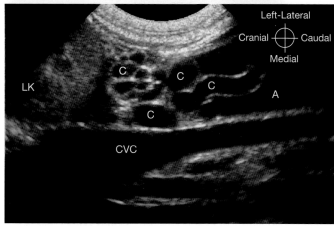

B

Figure 3.12   Acquired portosystemic (spleno-renal) collaterals. Compare with Fig 3.2A.

(A) Dilation of the left ovarian vein (LOV) results from acquired spleno-renal collaterals in a miniature schnauzer after partial attenuation of a congenital extrahepatic spleno-caval shunt. This color Doppler ultrasound image was made via the left flank with the dog in right lateral recumbency (plane 7). Arrows indicate the directions of blood flow. LRV – left renal vein; CVC – caudal vena cava. (Reproduced from Szatmári V et al. Ultrasonographic evaluation of partially attenuated congenital extrahepatic portosystemic shunts in 14 dogs. Vet Rec 2004; 155:448–456, with permission).

(B) Gray scale ultrasound image of spleno-renal acquired collaterals (C) caudal to the left kidney (LK) in a 1-year-old female Dutch schapendoes with sustained portal hypertension of hepatic origin. A – ascites; CVC – caudal vena cava. (Reproduced from Szatmári V et al. Ultrasonographic findings in dogs with hyperammonemia: 90 cases (2000-2002). J Am Vet Med Assoc 2004;224:717-727, with permission.)

Standard scanning planes for evaluating portal vein disorders

When a portal vein disorder is suspected, a routine abdominal ultrasound examination should be done and the abdominal vessels in all the following seven scanning planes should be examined.

Plane 1: left lateral recumbency, transverse intercostal section – the starting point

The transducer is placed in one of the last right intercostal spaces. One should find the intercostal space through which only the liver is seen without the right kidney, and the cross-sections of the aorta, the CVC and the PV are visualized. When the right kidney appears, the transducer should be angled cranially or moved to a more cranial intercostal space; when lungs that contain air appear, the transducer should be angled caudally or moved to a more caudal intercostal space. When the PV cannot be imaged because of duodenal gas, the transducer should be shifted dorsally within the same intercostal space and directed ventromedially.

Normal anatomy   From dorsal to ventral the cross-sections of the aorta, CVC and PV are seen; their cross-sectional areas are roughly equal (Fig. 3.14).

Congenital intrahepatic porto-caval shunts

The images do not differ from normal, except for the presence of a prominent hepatic artery between the CVC and PV. The hepatic artery is a pulsating

Figure 3.13 'Double caudal vena cava'. (Reproduced from Szatmári V et al. Ultrasonographic findings in dogs with hyperammonemia: 90 cases (2000–2002). J Am Vet Med Assoc 2004; 224:717–727, with permission.)
(A) Color Doppler ultrasound image of the left renal vein (LRV) as it enters the left common iliac vein (LCIV) in a 3-month-old female cairn terrier. Compare to Figure 3.12A! Dotted arrows indicate the direction of blood flow. The LCIV and RCIV fuse to form the CVC cranial to the LRV.
(B) Gray scale ultrasound image of the aortic trifurcation of the dog shown on Figure 3.13A. The left and right common iliac veins (LCIV, RCIV) run on the corresponding side of the aorta (AO). Plane 7, LEIA – left external iliac artery.

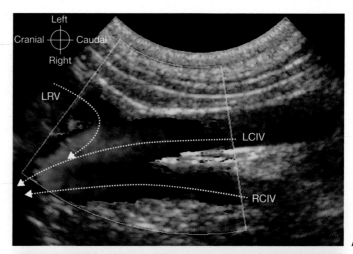

A

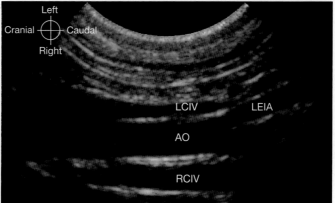

B

vessel with a smaller diameter compared to that of the PV.

Congenital extrahepatic spleno-caval, spleno-azygos, right gastric-caval and right gastric-azygos shunts
The PV is thinner than the aorta, sometimes to such an extent that it cannot even be recognized. The shunt might directly appear in this section.

Portal hypertension with APSCs
Visualization of the PV may often be hindered by ascitic fluid. If the PV is visible, the diameter is either smaller or larger compared to the aorta.

Plane 2: left lateral recumbency, transverse intercostal section – to image the right portal branch

Starting from plane 1, the PV is traced by angling or sliding the transducer cranially to the point

where the longitudinal image of the right portal branch appears.

Normal anatomy The right portal branch can consistently be found as a well-defined vein originating from the PV and running dorsolaterally to the right while becoming gradually thinner due to ramification (Fig. 3.15A).

Congenital intrahepatic porto-caval shunts
Each right-sided intrahepatic CPSS originates from the right portal branch as its direct continuation. The right portal branch is wide and does not taper to the periphery. The first segment of the shunt consistently runs dorsolaterally to the right, like a normal right portal branch, but then instead of ramification, it turns medially to enter the CVC (Fig. 3.15C,D). With little transducer-manipulation the entire course of the shunt can be traced to its caval termination.

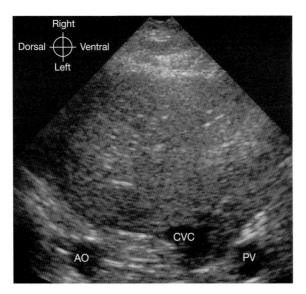

Figure 3.14 Normal great abdominal vessels. Gray scale ultrasound image of the liver of a healthy male adult beagle in plane 1 (i.e. transverse section via one of the last right intercostal spaces with the dog in left lateral recumbency). This is the starting point of the systematic ultrasound examination of the portal system. From dorsal to ventral the cross-sections of the aorta (AO), caudal vena cava (CVC) and portal vein (PV) are seen. The cross-sectional areas of the three vessels are approximately equal. (Reproduced from Szatmári V et al. Standard planes for ultrasonographic examination of the portal system in dogs. J Am Vet Med Assoc 2004; 224:713–716, with permission).

Figure 3.15 Right portal branch in 6 dogs. Plane 2, transverse section via a right intercostal space with the dog in left lateral recumbency to image the right portal branch.

(A) Normal right portal branch (PVbrR) at the point of its origin from the portal vein (PV) in a healthy adult male beagle. The right portal branch is thinner than the PV and becomes gradually thinner towards the periphery due to ramification. The right portal branch runs dorsolaterally and to the right. CVC – caudal vena cava. (Reproduced from Szatmári V et al. Standard planes for ultrasonographic examination of the portal system in dogs. J Am Vet Med Assoc 2004; 224:713–716, with permission).

(B) Color Doppler ultrasound image showing the right portal branch in a 1.5-year-old cairn terrier with a congenital extrahepatic spleno-caval shunt. The caudal vena cava (CVC) is easily recognizable, however at the site of the portal vein (PV) and right portal branch (PVbrR), only the walls of these collapsed vessels can be seen as hyperechoic structures. The color signs originate from the adjacent hepatic artery branch. HA – hepatic artery branch of the right lateral liver lobe; AO – aorta.

(C) Central divisional congenital porto-caval shunt. Gray scale ultrasound image of a 4-month-old male large mixed breed dog with a short intrahepatic porto-caval shunt (SH) that originates from the right portal branch (PVbrR). Compare the length of the shunt with the one shown in (D)! Three months after the surgical attenuation of this shunt the dog was euthanazed and a corrosion cast of the abdominal veins was made (see Fig. 3.6). CVC – caudal vena cava.

(D) Right divisional congenital intrahepatic portocaval shunt. Gray scale ultrasound image of an intrahepatic porto-caval shunt (SH) that originates from the right portal branch (PVbrR) in a 5.5-month-old male Labrador retriever. In this single image the direct connection between the right portal branch and the caudal vena cava (CVC) can be appreciated. The right portal branch is as wide as the portal vein (PV) and remains wide towards the periphery. (Reproduced from Szatmári V et al. Ultrasonographic findings in dogs with hyperammonemia: 90 cases (2000–2002). J Am Vet Med Assoc 2004; 224:717–727, with permission).

(E) Gray scale ultrasound image of the right portal branch (PVbrR) in a 5.5-month-old male Bernese mountain dog with an intrahepatic porto-caval shunt that originates from the left portal branch. The portal vein (PV) has a similar diameter to that of the caudal vena cava (CVC), however the right portal branch is very thin.

(F) Undetectable right portal branch of a dog with a left divisional congenital intrahepatic portocaval shunt. An artery is seen at the place where the right portal branch is expected. The localization and path of this vessel is compatible with a right portal branch, but the flow velocity is much higher in it (color aliasing). The hepatic artery and portal branches run adjacent to each other, but in this case the portal branch is undetectably thin. Dotted arrows indicate the direction of blood flow, CVC caudal – vena cava, HA – hepatic artery branch of the right lateral liver lobe, PV – portal vein.

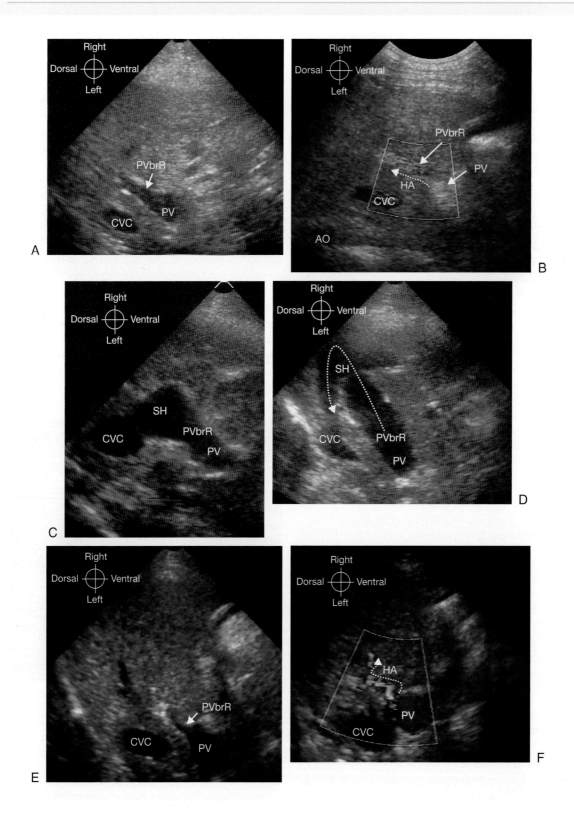

Left-sided intrahepatic CPSS must be suspected, when the findings described in plane 1 are compatible with an intrahepatic CPSS, and the right portal branch is absent or very thin in plane 2 (Fig. 3.15E). Often a hepatic artery branch is found at the place where the right portal branch is expected (Fig. 3.15F). On B-mode images this artery looks like a very thin right portal branch, but color Doppler mode reveals fast flow and pulsed wave Doppler mode shows arterial spectrum in it, confirming that it is a hepatic artery branch that runs adjacent to the hypoperfused right portal branch.

Congenital extrahepatic spleno-caval, spleno-azygos, right gastric-caval and right gastric-azygos shunts The right portal branch as well as the PV itself are usually so thin that they cannot be visualized either on B-mode or on color Doppler images (Fig. 3.15B).

Portal hypertension with APSCs The right portal branch can only be exceptionally visualized because of the ascites and small liver size. It can be thinner or wider than normal or might have a normal diameter corresponding to the diameter of the PV, and shows normal arborization, but undetectably slow flow (i.e. no color signals with the lowest possible PRF).

Plane 3: left lateral recumbency, transverse intercostal sections – to image congenital extrahepatic portosystemic shunts

Starting from plane 2, the transducer is gradually moved to caudal, keeping the PV and CVC in the image, to the level where the celiac artery originates from the aorta. Scanning should be performed first with B-mode, then repeated with color Doppler mode. The aim is to look for a direct connection between the PV and CVC, or for a vessel that originates from the PV with a hepatofugal flow direction.

Normal anatomy and congenital intrahepatic porto-caval shunts Immediately caudal to the portal bifurcation, the gastroduodenal vein may be imaged as it enters the ventral aspect of the PV from the right; however the gas-filled descending duodenum often hinders its visualization. Moving the transducer further caudally, the splenic vein can

be seen entering the left aspect of the PV from the ventrolateral direction. Slightly caudal to this point, the origins of the celiac and then the cranial mesenteric arteries from the aorta can be seen.

Congenital extrahepatic portosystemic shunts The origin of the cranial loop of the right gastric-caval shunts can sometimes be seen as hepatofugal flow in the gastroduodenal vein. However, the gastrointestinal gas often hinders their visualization. Therefore, plane 6 is recommended for use when a CPSS with a right gastric vein origin is suspected, based on the findings in planes 1, 2 and 3. The point where the shunt enters the CVC can usually be detected, but the course of the shunt loops can rarely be visualized from this side.

The entire length of spleno-caval shunts, and the origin of spleno-azygos shunts can always be visualized. Spleno-caval CPSSs make a short loop on the left side of the PV and CVC. The direct connection can usually be appreciated on B-mode images (Fig. 3.16), however occasionally, when the

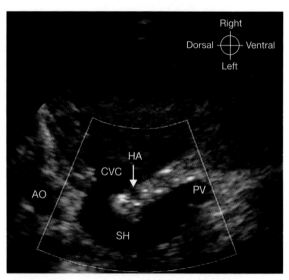

Figure 3.16 Congenital extrahepatic spleno-caval shunt. B-mode ultrasonogram showing the most common type of congenital portosystemic shunt in a 3.5-month-old female Jack Russell terrier in plane 3. Cross-sections of the aorta (AO), caudal vena cava (CVC) and portal vein (PV) are shown. Between the CVC and the PV the hepatic artery (HA) is seen. A short anomalous vein (SH) makes a direct connection between the PV and the CVC on their left side.

shunt does not appear on B-mode images because of insufficient gray scale resolution, color Doppler mode is helpful to visualize the shunt. Spleno-azygos shunts can be followed to the diaphragm.

Portal hypertension with APSCs Visualization of the PV is often difficult because of the presence of ascites. When the PV is imaged, it has a uniform diameter along its whole length. The origin of an APSC can occasionally be found as an anomalous vein with hepatofugal flow at the region where congenital extrahepatic spleno-caval shunts are expected to arise.

Plane 4: left lateral recumbency, longitudinal section via the right flank – to image the portal vein and the left divisional intrahepatic congenital portocaval shunts as well as the congenital extrahepatic portosystemic shunts

Longitudinal images of the PV and of the main portal branches are obtained with a transducer placed immediately caudal to the last rib and directed craniomedially. To find the PV, first the longitudinal image of the aorta should be obtained immediately ventral to the vertebrae. By ventral angulation of the transducer, the CVC becomes visible. Further ventral angulation results in the longitudinal image of the PV usually at the point where the splenic vein enters the PV. Firm transducer-pressure is often required to image the portal bifurcation.

In deep-chested and in large dogs the PV cannot usually be visualized via the right flank, hence an alternative approach is recommended, namely starting from plane 1 where the transducer should be rotated 90° to obtain a longitudinal image of the PV intercostally.

Normal anatomy The splenic vein can be seen to enter the PV from a caudolateral direction from the left (Fig. 3.1B). Tracing the PV cranially, the portal bifurcation can be seen with the wider left and the thinner right portal branch. Both branches become gradually thinner towards the periphery.

Congenital intrahepatic porto-caval shunts The PV at the level of the splenic vein looks similar to that of normal dogs. Tracing the PV cranially, an intrahepatic CPSS appears as the direct contin-

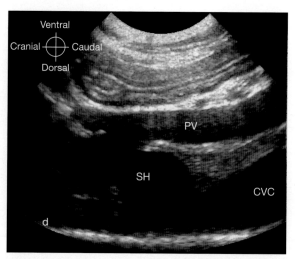

Figure 3.17 Patent ductus venosus. This intrahepatic porto-caval shunt originates from the left portal branch (i.e. left divisional shunt) in a 9-month-old hovawart. The portal trunk (PV) continues via a wide and tortuous anomalous vessel (SH) and terminates in the caudal vena cava (CVC). The image was made in plane 5. An empty stomach can be seen between the portal vein and the abdominal wall. Gas in the stomach would hinder the visualization of the shunt. d – diaphragm.

uation of the PV that enters the CVC. Plane 4 does not show the difference between intrahepatic CPSSs that originate from the right or left portal branch, however in plane 2, the right- and central-divisional intrahepatic CPSSs can be diagnosed and the left-divisional ones suspected. Plane 4 is used to confirm the presence of left-divisional intrahepatic CPSSs by direct visualization of the porto-caval connection (Fig. 3.17). Since the intrahepatic CPSSs that originate from the left portal branch run adjacent to the diaphragm, plane 4 allows better visualization of these than plane 2.

Congenital extrahepatic spleno–caval and spleno–azygos shunts Using plane 4, the PV segment that is cranial as well as caudal to the CPSS origin can also be seen in addition to the shunt, and the direction of flow can be determined (Fig. 3.7A). In cases of spleno-caval CPSSs, the termination of the CPSS can be found with a little transducer manipulation by tracing the shunting vessel. In cases of spleno-azygos shunts, the shunt can be traced to the point where it enters the thorax.

Occasionally the PV segment that is cranial to the point where the gastroduodenal vein enters the PV may also be imaged.

Congenital extrahepatic right gastric-caval and right gastric-azygos shunts Occasionally, the origin of the dilated right gastric vein can be visualized using this view, but not the path of the cranial loop of the shunt. The caudal shunt-loop (when it is present) can usually be visualized, originating at the same point as a congenital extrahepatic spleno-caval shunt, however it runs cranially, unlike a spleno-caval shunt which runs dorsally. The PV cranial to the origin of the caudal shunt loop can always be seen, and the flow direction is always hepatopetal in it. The anastomosis between the cranial and caudal loops of the shunt cannot be readily visualized with ultrasound, however the termination of the shunt can usually be found.

Portal hypertension with APSCs This view makes the assessment of portal flow velocity and of portal flow direction possible. The origin of APSCs arising from the PV may also be seen at the region where congenital extrahepatic spleno-caval shunts arise. It is usually impossible to image the PV cranial to the entering point of the gastroduodenal vein.

Plane 5: dorsal recumbency, longitudinal sections via the ventral abdominal wall – an alternative for plane 4

To find the PV in dorsal recumbency, the dog should be slightly tilted towards the sonologist. The right kidney and the caudate liver lobe are imaged first. The transducer is angled slightly ventro medially to image the CVC, then further medially to image the PV. To image the portal bifurcation, the PV is traced cranially. The transducer often has to be pushed firmly to move away the gas-filled intestinal loops.

The findings are the same as those described for plane 4, but in some cases plane 5 allows better visualization of the shunt or of the PV (Fig. 3.17), and provides better incidence angles for Doppler studies.

Plane-6: right lateral recumbency, longitudinal sections via the left flank – to image the (cranial loop of) congenital extrahepatic right gastric-caval and right gastric-azygos shunts

The transducer is placed immediately caudal to the last left rib and the PV is imaged longitudinally at the hilus of the liver. Finding the PV using this approach is difficult and is only necessary when in plane 3, an extrahepatic CPSS is suspected but its entire visualization is impossible.

Another way to find the right gastric-caval shunts is to follow the hepatic artery from its origin to the liver, as the hepatic artery crosses the cranial shunt loop. To find the hepatic artery, the celiac artery has to be imaged as it originates from the aorta, cranial to the left kidney.[32] The hepatic artery is the widest branch of the celiac artery, which runs cranially to the liver between the PV and the CVC. Color Doppler mode helps to find the hepatic artery when the gray scale resolution is insufficient to visualize this thin vessel. The color signals of the hepatic artery indicate higher flow velocity compared to that of the CVC and the PV.

Congenital extrahepatic right gastric-caval or right gastric-azygos shunts Usually, when the PV is being investigated, a large-caliber anomalous vein (i.e. the shunt) appears just under the body wall, even before the PV is actually found. The diameter of this CPSS is comparable to that of the CVC. Tracing the shunt cranially it seems to originate from the PV, at the hilus of the liver (Fig. 3.11A). From its origin, the shunt should be traced to its termination, with and also without color Doppler mode (Fig. 3.11B). The PV cranial to the shunt origin is too thin to be visualized.

Normal anatomy, congenital intrahepatic porto-caval shunts, congenital extrahepatic spleno-caval and spleno-azygos shunts, and portal hypertension with APSCs The large-caliber anomalous vein described above is absent. The normal right gastric vein is so thin that it cannot be visualized ultrasonographically.

Plane 7: right lateral recumbency, longitudinal sections via the left flank – to image the dilated left gonadal vein, i.e. the termination of acquired spleno-renal collaterals

The CVC is imaged in longitudinal section by placing the transducer immediately ventral to the lumbar vertebrae and caudal to the left kidney. Keeping the longitudinal image of the CVC, the transducer is moved cranially to image the left renal vein as it enters the CVC. With B- and color Doppler modes a vein has to be searched that enters the dilated left renal vein from the caudal aspect: this is the left gonadal vein.

Normal anatomy, congenital intra- and extra-hepatic portosystemic shunts   Caudal to the left kidney, two great vessels, namely the aorta and the CVC can be seen running parallel to each other; the aorta is located more to the left. The left gonadal vein can never be visualized because it is too thin. The left renal artery (occasionally double) runs adjacent to the left renal vein and can be differentiated from the vein even on gray scale images by its smaller diameter and pulsation.

Portal hypertension with APSCs   The dilated left gonadal vein can always be seen entering the left renal vein from the caudal aspect (Figs 3.2A, 3.12A), except in cases of tense ascites, when not even the CVC can be visualized. When the left gonadal vein is very wide, it appears as a third great vessel on the left side of the aorta. This image has to be carefully differentiated from a 'double CVC'. Several small tortuous veins (spleno-renal collaterals) may often, but not always be seen around the left renal vein (Fig. 3.12B).

Summary

Ultrasonography is a highly sensitive and specific, non-invasive diagnostic method to diagnose and exclude CPSSs and APSCs in non-sedated dogs. The exclusion of portosystemic shunting is not only based on the fact that no anomalous veins can be found, but also on the fact that the morphological and hemodynamic features of the abdominal vessels are different in dogs with normal vascular anatomy from those with portal vein disorders. The diagnosis of a particular portal venous disorder is the result of a puzzle that is based on the results of clinical, laboratory, histopathologic and ultrasonographic findings.

SPECIFIC FEATURES OF FELINE PORTAL VEIN ANOMALIES

Portal vein disorders occur much less frequently in cats than in dogs, and there are several differences in the etiology of APSCs and in the anatomy of the CPSSs and APSCs. This short chapter will focus only on these differences. The scanning technique recommended for cats is the same as that used for dogs (i.e. the seven standard planes), but the findings and their interpretation may be different.

Etiology of feline hyperammonemia

High blood ammonia levels in cats can be caused by CPSS, APSCs and by arginine deficiency.[33,34] Arginine deficiency develops in anorectic cats along with hepatic lipidosis, which can be diagnosed with abdominal ultrasonography and cytology of a hepatic fine needle aspiration biopsy.[35] Urea cycle enzyme deficiency has not been reported in the cat.

Routine abdominal ultrasound examination often reveals no abnormalities in cats with CPSS or with APSC due to intrahepatic portal hypertension. Ascites is absent not only in cats with CPSS, but usually also in cats with APSCs; the liver and kidneys are usually of normal size in both. Splenomegaly may be present in cats with portal hypertension.

Portal hypertension in cats

Acquired portosystemic collaterals can develop as a result of intra- or prehepatic portal hypertension. Prehepatic portal hypertension can be caused by an obstruction of the PV by a thrombus or by a compression by a tumor.[33] Congenital arterioportal fistula has also been found as the cause of APSCs.[33,36] Intrahepatic portal hypertension is often the result of hepatic fibrosis which is often caused by congenital hepatic fibrosis due to polycystic kidney and liver disease (PKD).[33,37,38] Free abdominal fluid is either absent, or if it is present, the amount is very small.

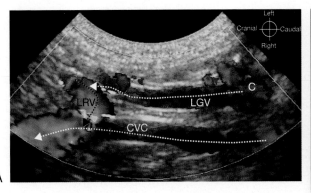
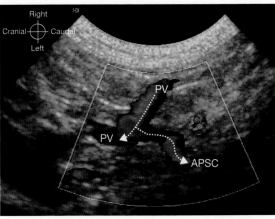

Figure 3.18 Feline portal hypertension. Ultrasonographic signs of portal hypertension are shown in a 3-year-old female British short hair cat due to congenital hepatic fibrosis on the basis of polycystic kidney and liver disease. No renal cysts were seen with ultrasonography in this cat. Dotted arrows indicate the direction of blood flow.
(A) The left gonadal vein (LGV) becomes dilated when spleno-renal collateral circulation develops. Color Doppler image made in plane 7. CVC – caudal vena cava, LRV – left renal vein, C – conglomeration of portosystemic collateral vessels. Compare to Fig. 3.12A.
(B) Color Doppler ultrasound image of the portal vein (PV) and the origin of an acquired portosystemic collateral vein (APSC) made in plane 4. CA – celiac artery. Compare to Fig. 3.3A.

Acquired portosystemic collaterals in cats

The anatomy of feline APSCs is slightly different from that of the dog.[39–41] As spleno-renal collaterals do not develop consistently, the left gonadal vein may not be dilated.[33] When spleno-renal collaterals do develop, a dilated left gonadal vein will be present, similar to dogs (Fig. 3.18A). However, a sort of extrahepatic CPSS terminates in the left renal vein mimicking a dilated left gonadal vein. The difference is that in the case of a dilated left gonadal vein (i.e. APSCs) color Doppler usually reveals lots of small tortuous veins around the gonadal vein, and the left gonadal vein cannot be followed to the PV because it ends in a conglomeration of small collaterals. In contrast, a CPSS that enters the left renal vein is a very wide vein (wider than the CVC) and can be traced back to its PV origin (Fig. 3.20).

The origin of an APSC is often found starting directly from the PV at the point where congenital extrahepatic spleno-caval shunts originate in dogs, i.e. slightly cranial to the point where the celiac artery originates from the aorta (Fig. 3.18B). Color Doppler mode may reveal hepatofugal, hepatopetal or zero flow in the PV cranial to the collateral origin. This APSC runs in the caudal direction and tends to disappear among the intestines.

When the presence of APSCs is suspected, ultrasound-guided biopsy of the liver should be taken for histopathological examination. Suspicion should be especially strong when renal cysts have been detected or when an abnormal abdominal vein in a Persian or British short hair breed or their crosses has been found.

Congenital portosystemic shunts in cats

In contrast to dogs, CPSSs in cats have a great anatomical variety.[4,42] The shunting vessel is usually a single extrahepatic wide vein.

Intrahepatic CPSSs

Intrahepatic CPSSs are very rare in cats and unlike in dogs, they are not necessarily the continuations of the left or right portal branches, therefore they may be fairly thin.

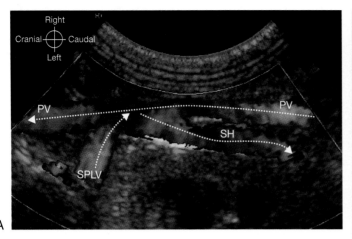

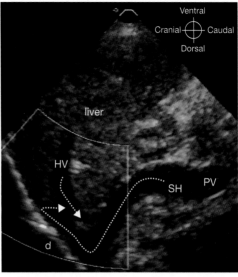

Figure 3.19 Congenital extrahepatic portosystemic shunts in two cats. Dotted arrows indicate the direction of blood flow.

(A) The shunt (SH) of this European short hair cat originates directly from the portal vein (PV) just caudal to the point where the splenic vein (SPLV) enters the PV. Interestingly, the PV does not become thinner cranial to the shunt origin and it displays hepatopetal flow. This color Doppler image was made in plane 4. Compare to Fig. 3.7A.

(B) The extrahepatic shunt (SH) of this Maine coon cat seems to be intrahepatic, but surgery revealed that it actually ran between the liver lobes. The shunt connects the portal vein (PV) and a hepatic vein (HV). This B-mode image was made in plane 5. d – diaphragm.

Extrahepatic CPSSs

Feline spleno-caval and spleno-azygos shunts are similar to those in dogs, however the shunt may originate directly from the PV adjacent to the point where the splenic vein enters the PV (Fig. 3.19A). If the shunt originates more caudally from the PV then hepatofugal flow can often be seen in the PV segment between the shunt origin and the entry point of the splenic vein. However, the blood flow may be hepatopetal in the entire PV. The PV may get thinner cranial to the origin of a CPSS, but may have a uniform diameter throughout its whole length.

Extrahepatic CPSSs arising from the right gastric vein are rather common in dogs, but do not occur in cats. However, there are two types of CPSSs that are quite specific for the cat. One originates slightly caudal to the portal bifurcation and runs cranially among liver lobes along the esophagus and eventually enters the CVC (often via a hepatic vein) between the diaphragmatic surface of the liver and the diaphragm. Ultrasonographically this shunt appears to be intrahepatic because the vessel is surrounded by liver (Fig. 3.19B). The other type of CPSS originates from the cranial mesenteric vein or from the PV at the region where it is formed from the mesenteric veins. From here the wide shunting vessel runs caudally along the colon as far backwards as caudal to the aortic trifurcation, where it makes a 180° turn and runs cranially on the left side of the CVC, terminating in the left renal vein or in the CVC caudal to the left kidney (Fig. 3.20). This type of CPSS can easily be found using plane 7, and should be carefully differentiated from a dilated left gonadal vein which is the result of spleno-renal APSCs.

Acknowledgments

The photographs were supplied by Mr Aart van der Woude and Mr Joop Fama. The corrosion casts were made with the help of Mr Richard Lenters and Mr Wim Kersten.

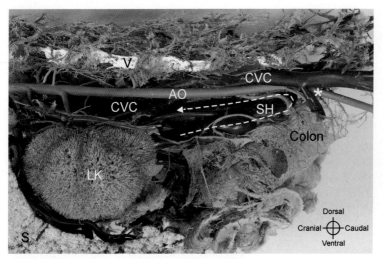

Figure 3.20 Congenital extrahepatic portosystemic shunt in a cat. Corrosion cast of the abdominal blood vessels of a kitten with a congenital extrahepatic portocaval shunt. The veins are blue and the arteries are green. The shunt (SH) is a wide vessel that runs caudal from its origin (cranial mesenteric vein) along the descending colon (Colon). At the level of the aortic trifurcation (*) the SH turns back in the cranial direction and runs on the left side of the caudal vena cava (CVC) to eventually terminate in the CVC slightly caudal to the left kidney (LK). AO – aorta, S – spleen, V – vertebrae.

References

1. Evans HE. The heart and arteries. In: Evans HE, ed. Miller's anatomy of the dog. 3rd edn. Philadelphia: WB Saunders; 1993:586–681.
2. Evans HE. The veins. In: Evans HE, ed. Miller's anatomy of the dog. 3rd edn. Philadelphia: WB Saunders; 1993:682–716.
3. Vitums A. Portal vein in the dog. Zbl Vet Med 1959; 7:723-741.
4. Van den Ingh TSGAM, Rothuizen J, Meyer HP. Circulatory disorders of the liver in dogs and cats. Vet Q 1995; 17:70–76.
5. Vitums A. Portosystemic communications in the dog. Acta Anat (Basel) 1959; 39:271–299.
6. Johnson SE. Portal hypertension. Part I. Pathophysiology and clinical consequences. Comp Cont Educ Pract Vet 1987; 9:741–748.
7. Sterczer Á, Meyer HP, Boswijk HC, Rothuizen J. Evaluation of ammonia measurements in dogs with two analysers for use in veterinary practice. Vet Rec 1999; 144:523–526.
8. Rothuizen J, van den Ingh TSGAM. Rectal ammonia tolerance test in the evaluation of portal circulation in dogs with liver disease. Res Vet Sci 1982; 33:22–25.
9. Szatmári V, Rothuizen J, van den Ingh TSGAM, et al. Ultrasonographic findings in dogs with hyperammonemia: 90 cases (2000–2002). J Am Vet Med Assoc 2004; 224:717–727.
10. Strombeck DR, Meyer DJ, Freedlan RA. Hyperammonemia due to a urea cycle enzyme deficiency in two dogs. J Am Vet Med Assoc 1975; 166:1109–1111.
11. Wrigley RH, Konde LJ, Park RD, et al. Ultrasonographic diagnosis of portacaval shunts in young dogs. J Am Vet Med Assoc 1987; 191:421–424.
12. Tiemessen I, Rothuizen J, Voorhout G. Ultrasonography in the diagnosis of congenital portosystemic shunts in dogs. Vet Q 1995; 17:50–53.
13. Lamb CR. Ultrasonographic diagnosis of congenital portosystemic shunts in dogs: results of a prospective study. Vet Radiol Ultrasound 1996; 37:281–288.
14. Wolschrijn CF, Mahapokai W, Rothuizen J, et al. Gauged attenuation of congenital portosystemic shunts: results in 160 dogs and 15 cats. Vet Q 2000; 22:94–98.
15. Szatmári V, Rothuizen J, Voorhout G. Standard planes for ultrasonographic examination of the portal system in dogs. J Am Vet Med Assoc 2004; 224:713–716.
16. Szatmári V, Németh T, Kótai I, et al. Doppler ultrasonographic diagnosis and anatomy of congenital arterioportal fistula in a puppy. Vet Radiol Ultrasound 2000; 41:284–286.
17. Sterczer Á, Gaál T, Perge E, et al. Chronic hepatitis in the dog – a review. Vet Q 2001; 23:148–152.
18. Boomkens SY, Penning LC, Egberink HF, et al. Hepatitis with special reference to dogs. A review on the pathogenesis and infectious etiologies, including unpublished results of recent own studies. Vet Q 2004; 26:107–114.
19. Van den Ingh TSGAM, Rothuizen J. Lobular dissecting hepatitis in juvenile and young adult dogs. J Vet Intern Med 1994; 8:217–220.

20. Van den Ingh TSGAM, Rothuizen J, Meyer HP. Portal hypertension associated with primary hypoplasia of the hepatic portal vein in dogs. Vet Rec 1995; 137:424–427.
21. Szatmári V. Simultaneous congenital and acquired extrahepatic portosystemic shunts in two dogs – letter to the editor. Vet Radiol Ultrasound 2003; 44:486–487.
22. Szatmári V, Rothuizen J, van Sluijs FJ, et al. Ultrasonographic evaluation of partially attenuated congenital extrahepatic portosystemic shunts in 14 dogs. Vet Rec 2004; 155:448–456.
23. Meyer HP, Rothuizen J, van den Brom WE, et al. Quantitation of portosystemic shunting in dogs by ultrasound-guided injection of 99MTc-macroaggregates into a splenic vein. Res Vet Sci 1994; 57:58–62.
24. Rothuizen J, van den Ingh TSGAM, Voorhout G, et al. Congenital porto-systemic shunts in sixteen dogs and three cats. J Small Anim Pract 1982; 23:67–81.
25. Lamb CR, White RN. Morphology of congenital intrahepatic portocaval shunts in dogs and cats. Vet Rec 1998; 142:55–60.
26. Hunt GB, Youmans KR, Sommerlad S, et al. Surgical management of multiple congenital intrahepatic shunts in two dogs: case report. Vet Surg 1998; 27:262–267.
27. Favier RP, Szatmári V, Rothuizen J. Multiple congenital portal vein anomalies in a dog. Vet Rec 2004; 154:604–605.
28. Hunt GB, Bellenger CR, Borg R, et al. Congenital interruption of the portal vein and caudal vena cava in dogs: six case reports and a review of the literature. Vet Surg 1998; 27:203–215.
29. Hall JA, Allen TA, Fettman MJ. Hyperammonemia associated with urethral obstruction in a dog. J Am Vet Med Assoc 1987; 191:1116–1118.
30. Meyer HP, Rothuizen J, Tiemessen I, et al. Transient metabolic hyperammonaemia in young Irish Wolfhounds. Vet Rec 1996; 138:105–107.
31. Laborda J, Gimeno M, Dominguez L, et al. Anomalous caudal vena cava in the dog. Vet Rec 1996; 138:20–21.
32. Szatmári V, Sótonyi P, Vörös K. Normal duplex Doppler waveforms of the major abdominal blood vessels in dogs: a review. Vet Radiol Ultrasound 2001; 42:93–107.
33. Szatmári V, van den Ingh TSGAM, Rothuizen J. Ultrasonographic diagnosis of acquired portosystemic collaterals in six cats. Abstract. 14th ECVIM congress, Barcelona, Spain, September 9–11, 2004: 207.
34. Morris JG, Rogers QR. Ammonia intoxication in the near-adult cat as a result of a dietary deficiency of arginine. Science 1978; 199:431–432.
35. Center SA. Feline hepatic lipidosis. Vet Clin North Am Small Anim Pract 2005; 35:225–269.
36. Legender AM, Krahwinkel DJ, Carrig CB, et al. Ascites associated with intrahepatic arteriovenous fistula in a cat. J Am Vet Med Assoc 1976; 168:589–591.
37. Bosje JT, van den Ingh TSGAM, van der Linde-Sipman JS. Polycystic kidney and liver disease in cats. Vet Q 1998; 20:136–139.
38. Zanduliet MMJM, Szatmári V, van den Ingh TSGAM, Rothuizen J. Acquired portosystemic shunting in 2 cats secondary to congenital hepatic fibrosis. J Vet Int Med 2005; 19:765–767.
39. Vitums A. Portosystemic communications in animals with hepatic cirrhosis and malignant lymphoma. J Am Vet Med Assoc 1961; 138;31–34.
40. Khan IR, Vitums A. Portosystemic communications in the cat. Res Vet Sci 1971; 12:215–218.
41. Inglés AC, Légaré DJ, Lautt WW. Development of portocaval shunts in portal-stenotic cats. Can J Physiol Pharmacol 1993; 71:671–674.
42. Lamb CR, Forster-van Hijfte MA, White RN, et al. Ultrasonographic diagnosis of congenital portosystemic shunt in 14 cats. J Small Anim Pract 1996; 37:205–209.

Chapter 4

Morphological classification of circulatory disorders of the canine and feline liver

John M. Cullen, Ted S. G. A. M. van den Ingh, Susan E. Bunch,
Jan Rothuizen, Robert J. Washabau, Valeer J. Desmet

CHAPTER CONTENTS

INTRODUCTION

For the recognition of the lesions associated with the various circulatory disorders in dogs and cats, it is essential to understand the normal hepatic circulation, and to know the consequences of impaired hepatic perfusion as well as the histological pattern of portal venous hypoperfusion. The circulatory disorders of the liver in dogs and cats can be categorized as congenital portosystemic shunts, disorders associated with outflow disturbances resulting in passive congestion, and disorders associated with portal hypertension.

The diagnosis of most of the circulatory diseases does not depend on histological evaluation of the liver. For congenital portosystemic shunts, ultrasonography is the diagnostic method of choice as explained in detail in Chapter 3. Arterioportal shunts are also diagnosed by ultrasonography. Primary portal vein hypoplasia, however, should be diagnosed on the basis of negative ultrasonography of the portal vasculature and the typical but nonspecific findings of histology of the liver. Blood tests to find or exclude portosystemic collateral circulation (either acquired due to portal hypertension or due to congenital portosystemic shunts) are the plasma bile acid and ammonia concentration. Functional testing can be performed by postprandial bile acid measurement or ammonia tolerance test (rectal or oral), respectively. Finally, there are several scintigraphic techniques using

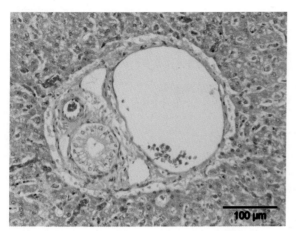

Figure 4.1 Dog. Portal area with normal profiles of the portal vein, hepatic artery and bile duct. Dilated lymphatics. HE.

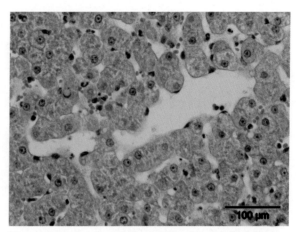

Figure 4.2 Cat. Terminal hepatic vein with draining sinusoids. HE.

[99]mTechnetium to demonstrate or quantify portosystemic shunting. The critical diagnostic steps of the vascular disorders of the liver are summarized in Table 4.1 at the end of the chapter.

NORMAL HEPATIC CIRCULATION

The liver is supplied with blood by the hepatic artery and the portal vein. The portal vein drains the splanchnic viscera, i.e. stomach, intestine, spleen and pancreas, and normally contributes to approximately 70% of the total hepatic blood flow.[1] The portal vein is formed by the confluence of cranial and caudal mesenteric veins and receives the splenic and gastroduodenal vein before it enters the liver at the porta hepatis.[2,3] Here the portal vein divides into a short right branch and a large left branch. The right branch serves the right side of the liver whereas the left branch serves the left and central divisions of the liver. They then subdivide into successively smaller branches.[4] The intrahepatic portal vein branches are situated in the portal areas and represent by far the largest structure in the portal areas (Fig. 4.1). The terminal branches, present in the smallest portal areas, finally give rise to the inlet venules which penetrate the periportal limiting plate and open into the sinusoids. The hepatic artery accompanies the portal vein and two or more branches may be present within each portal area. The terminal distribution of the arteries is by three routes, i.e. the periportal plexus,

which is characteristically distributed around portal vein branches within the portal area, the peribiliary plexus, which supplies all the intrahepatic bile ducts, and the terminal hepatic artery branches, which have an internal elastic lamina and a layer of smooth muscle cells and open directly into periportal sinusoids.[1] The hepatic artery also supplies the Glisson's capsule and some arteries supply the hepatic venous plexus surrounding the larger draining hepatic veins. From the sinusoids the blood enters directly into the terminal hepatic veins (synonym: central veins) (Fig. 4.2). Sphincters in the wall of these arterioles, in the inlet venules and at the outlet of the sinusoids to the hepatic veins regulate the acinar microcirculation and hence probably parenchymal function.[1] The terminal hepatic veins unite to form the intercalated or sublobular veins which in turn anastomose to form the large hepatic veins which finally drain into the caudal caval vein. In dogs, the sublobular or intercalated hepatic veins are characterized by a relatively thin wall with a spiral shaped smooth muscle and are surrounded by loosely structured stromal tissue (Fig. 4.3),[5] whereas in cats they are characterized by a relatively thick fibrous wall (Fig. 4.4).

While the portal vein supplies the larger amount of blood to the liver, the liver is not capable of directly controlling this flow and changes in flow within the portal vein are largely determined by factors affecting intestinal blood flow. So, hepatic blood flow increases after feeding and decreases

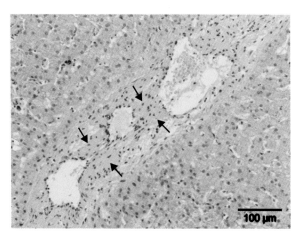

Figure 4.3 Dog. Normal sublobular hepatic vein characterized by a relatively thin wall with a spiral shaped smooth muscle (arrows) and surrounded by loosely structured stromal tissue. HE.

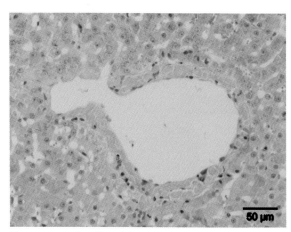

Figure 4.4 Cat. Transition of the terminal hepatic vein to the sublobular hepatic vein which is characterized by a relatively thick fibrous wall. HE.

during sleep and exercise. Total hepatic blood flow is regulated by hepatic artery autoregulation, which means that if portal flow increases, arterial flow will decrease, and vice-versa.[6,7]

Although the liver normally produces large quantities of lymph fluid, lymph vessels are not easily seen under normal conditions. With increased lymph production dilated lymphatics can be observed at three possible locations, i.e. in the portal areas (Fig. 4.1), around the larger hepatic veins and in the Glisson's capsule. Lymph vessels, however, do not exist in the hepatic parenchyma due to the peculiar structure of the hepatic sinusoids.[1]

In fetal life the umbilical vein contributes markedly to the afferent hepatic flow; it usually communicates with the portal vein where the portal vein divides into the (intralobular) veins of the left central and lateral liver lobes. Most umbilical blood is directed towards the ductus venosus, a fetal connection between the portal vein and the posterior caval vein situated opposite the inflow opening of the umbilical vein.[4] Thus the umbilical blood directly streams into the posterior caval vein, bypassing the sinusoidal vascular bed of the liver. After birth the ductus venosus closes by sphincteric contraction and subsequently disappears. Functional closure occurs within 3 days, whereas structural closure takes 15–18 days in the dog.[8] The

remnant structure of the umbilical vein becomes the ligamentum teres hepatis (synonym: round ligament).

CONSEQUENCES OF IMPAIRED HEPATIC PERFUSION

The function of the liver is highly dependent on adequate perfusion and hence malperfusion may cause gross and microscopic pathological changes in the liver and clinical disease.

Hepatic atrophy

Maintenance of the mass and function of the hepatic parenchyma is largely determined by hepatic perfusion, particularly by the quantity and quality of the portal blood. This contains many nutrients and specific hepatotrophic factors. Lack of nutrients and hepatotrophic factors in the portal blood, e.g. in cachexia, or deprivation of these factors by reduced portal blood flow, leads to atrophy (of the deprived segment) of the liver. Regionally decreased perfusion of the liver (e.g. thrombosis of the left branch of the portal vein) often results in increased hepatic blood flow and hypertrophy of the remaining (right) part of the liver (Fig. 4.5).[9]

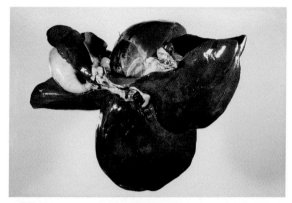

Figure 4.5 Dog. Left-sided atrophy of the liver due to thrombosis of the left branch of the portal vein and compensatory hypertrophy of the right side of the liver.

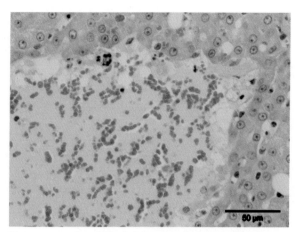

Figure 4.7 Cat. Peliosis: parenchymal type. HE.

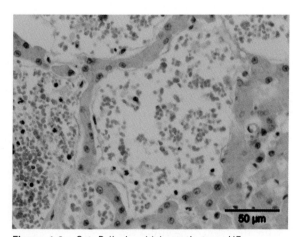

Figure 4.6 Cat. Peliosis: phlebectatic type. HE.

Peliosis hepatis

Peliosis hepatis is defined as randomly distributed, cystic blood-filled spaces in the liver; it occurs rarely in dogs and is more common in cats.[10,11] These may result from local obstruction of small branches of the portal vein with subsequent focal hepatic atrophy and sinusoidal dilatation (phlebectatic type, also called teleangiectasis (Fig. 4.6)), or from focal hepatocytic necrosis (parenchymal type) (Fig. 4.7). A strict division in these two types may not be as clear as suggested above as both types can be seen in the same animals.[11] They may even have an identical pathogenesis whereby the phlebectatic type represents a more slowly developing lesion with focal portal venous hypoperfusion, and the parenchymal type an acute and more severe obstructive and ischaemic lesion (vide infra). Teleangiectasis associated with prolonged use of steroids, as observed in humankind, has an unknown pathogenesis and until now has not been observed in dogs and cats.

Ischemic hepatic necrosis

The parenchyma of the liver is protected against ischemia by its double blood supply and, in the healthy dog, the liver can survive complete loss of perfusion by either the portal vein or the hepatic artery without infarction.

Infarction of the liver

Infarction of the liver occurs infrequently and usually results from either combined obstruction of the hepatic artery and the portal vein, or from obstruction of the portal vein or the hepatic artery in combination with hepatic vein obstruction. The subsequent acute ischemia causes hepatic necrosis. Infarcts tend to occur at the margins of the liver and are recognized microscopically without magnification, as sharply delineated pale or dark red areas (Fig. 4.8).[12,13]

Generalized centrolobular ischemic necrosis

Generalized centrolobular ischemic necrosis is much more common (Fig. 4.9) and occurs with

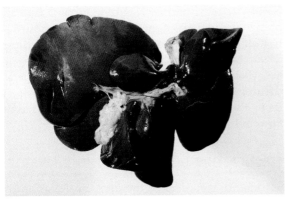

Figure 4.8 Dog. Multiple pale well-delineated infarcts at the margins of the liver.

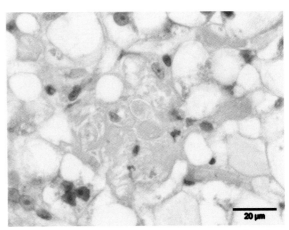

Figure 4.10 Dog. Focal ischemic necrosis associated with disseminated intravascular coagulation and thrombus formation in the sinusoids. HE.

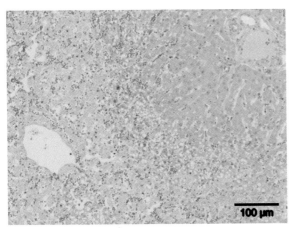

Figure 4.9 Cat. Generalized centrolobular ischemic necrosis associated with acute cardiac decompensation (cardiac shock). HE.

(cardiac) shock when arterial flow and portal vein oxygen saturation are decreased simultaneously or with severe (acute) anemia.[14]

Focal ischemic necrosis

Focal ischemic necrosis is particularly associated with disseminated intravascular coagulation and associated focal thrombotic obstruction of sinusoids with subsequent ischemic necrosis of adjacent hepatocytes (Fig. 4.10).

HISTOLOGICAL PATTERN OF PORTAL VEIN HYPOPERFUSION

One of the principal challenges for pathologists trying to diagnose vascular disorders of the liver is the stereotypical histological response of the liver to inadequate portal vein flow (Fig. 4.11). With decreased portal blood flow, the profile of the portal vein in the portal tracts becomes diminished or absent. Hepatic arteries respond to hypoperfusion of the liver and increase their blood flow.[6,7] As a result they become more tortuous and hypertrophied and/or may proliferate. Histologically, this produces an increased number of arteriolar profiles in the portal tracts and probably makes formerly non-apparent intralobular arterioles more prominent. Sometimes, an increased number of ductular profiles and slight portal fibrosis may also occur. Additional changes in the parenchyma that may be seen are hepatocellular atrophy, the presence of lipogranulomas and sinusoidal dilatation, particularly in the periportal areas. The latter is probably the result of the increased arterial hepatic flow with focal increased sinusoidal pressure and subsequent sinusoidal dilatation.

The classic example of this stereotypical reaction of portal vein hypoperfusion in the dog is the Eck's fistula, an experimental surgically produced portocaval shunt (Fig. 4.12). Similar lesions are seen in various circulatory disorders associated with portal venous hypoperfusion such as congenital

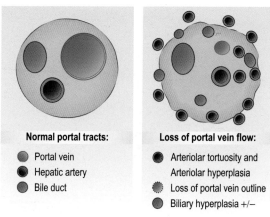

Normal portal tracts:

- Portal vein
- Hepatic artery
- Bile duct

Loss of portal vein flow:

- Arteriolar tortuosity and Arteriolar hyperplasia
- Loss of portal vein outline
- Biliary hyperplasia +/−

Figure 4.11   Schematic presentation of stereotypical response of the liver to portal vein hypoperfusion. Changes in the portal areas are most prominent and shown here are: small or invisible portal vein branch, multiple cross-sections of tortuous and hyperplastic hepatic artery branches, and sometimes biliary hyperplasia. Parenchymal changes may be hepatocellular atrophy, the presence of lipogranulations, and sinusoidal dilatation particularly in the periportal areas.

portosystemic shunts, arterioportal fistulas, primary hypoplasia of the portal vein, and obstruction of the portal vein (vide infra). Some of these characteristics also may be seen in primary chronic liver diseases associated with portal hypertension as cirrhosis or congenital hepatic fibrosis, in which there also exists persistent decreased portal blood flow and increased hepatic arterial flow.

CIRCULATORY DISORDERS OF THE LIVER

Circulatory disorders of the liver can be grouped into three major categories: congenital portosystemic shunts, disorders with outflow disturbances resulting in passive congestion of the liver, and disorders associated with deranged inflow of portal blood and portal hypertension. Histological examination of liver biopsies can aid in the diagnosis of all of these disorders, but due to considerable overlap in the appearance of several of these conditions, additional clinical, biochemical, or imaging information may be needed to formulate a final diagnosis. The relationship of the different procedures needed to make a diagnosis is summarized in Table 4.1 at the end of the chapter.

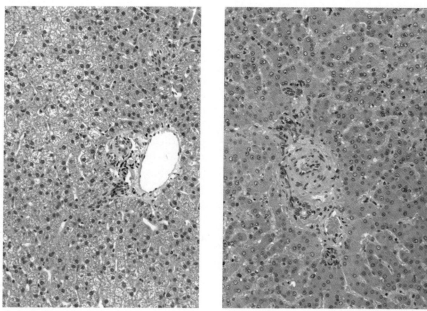

A   B

Figure 4.12   Dog, Eck's fistula. Preoperative (A) normal aspect of the portal area and postoperative (B) aspect with loss of portal vein profile and proliferation of arterioles. HE.

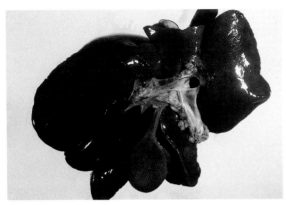

Figure 4.13 Dog. Congenital intrahepatic portosystemic shunt originating from the right branch of the portal vein.

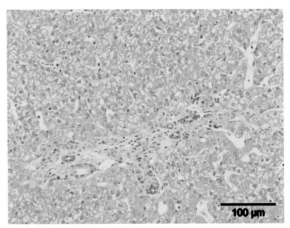

Figure 4.14 Dog. Congenital portosystemic shunt. Portal area without recognizable portal vein and arteriolar proliferation. Some dilated sinusoids in the hepatic parenchyma. HE.

Congenital portosystemic shunts

Congenital portosystemic shunts (CPSSs) are single large calibre vascular anomalies that directly connect the portal venous system with the systemic venous circulation. CPSSs are more frequently seen in dogs than in cats. They may be intrahepatic or extrahepatic. Intrahepatic shunts result from a failure of the ductus venosus to close after birth. They mostly originate from the left branch of the portal vein, which is consistent with the normal embryology of the ductus venosus. Sometimes they originate from the right branch of the portal vein and drain directly into the posterior caval vein (Fig. 4.13). Extrahepatic shunts represent abnormal functional communications; they may arise from any part of the portal system and may drain in the caudal caval vein or the (hemi)azygos vein. In the dog most extrahepatic shunts originate at the junction of the splenic and the left gastric vein. The shunt may receive its main volume of blood directly from the splenic vein, or from the gastro-duodenal vein via the communicating right and left gastric vein. The drainage site at the caudal caval vein is usually situated between the phrenico-abdominal vein and the liver. In the dog, intra-hepatic shunts are most often seen in large breeds, whereas in small breeds the shunts are usually extrahepatic. In the cat both intrahepatic and extra-hepatic shunts occur; extrahepatic shunts vary widely with respect to their origin and course.[9]

The pathological changes of CPSSs are secondary to the shunting of blood past the liver. Macro-

scopic changes are liver atrophy, and when there is an extrahepatic shunt, hypoplasia of the portal vein downstream from the origin of the shunt. The degree of change in the hepatic histology is probably a function of the amount of portal blood that is diverted from the liver and may vary between liver lobes depending on the site of the shunt vessel, particularly with intrahepatic shunts. The histological changes are characteristic for portal venous hypoperfusion (vide supra) and consist of loss of portal vein profiles, increased numbers of arteriolar profiles, hepatocellular atrophy with lipogranulomas and sometimes periportal sinusoidal dilatation (Figs 4.14, 4.15). The histological appearance of affected cats and dogs is similar.

An important clinical feature of this disorder is that portal hypertension does not occur.

Disorders associated with outflow disturbances affecting the heart, caudal vena cava or the hepatic veins

Impairment of venous outflow results in passive congestion of the liver. Passive congestion of the liver is characterized by engorgement and dilatation of the hepatic veins and centrilobular sinusoids (Fig. 4.16), and sometimes extravasation of erythrocytes in the liver cell plates (Fig. 4.17). In these areas there will be atrophy and subsequent loss of hepatocytes as well as gradual development of

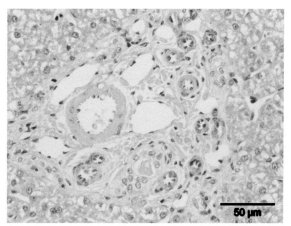

Figure 4.15 Dog. Congenital portosystemic shunt. Portal area without recognizable portal vein, arteriolar proliferation, dilated lymphatics. HE.

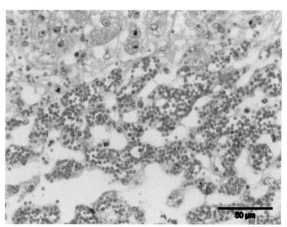

Figure 4.17 Cat. Acute passive congestion. Extravasation of erythrocytes in the liver cell plates with loss of the hepatocytes. HE.

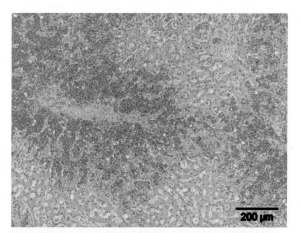

Figure 4.16 Dog. Passive congestion. Centrolobular engorgement and dilatation of the sinusoids with atrophy of the hepatic cords. HE.

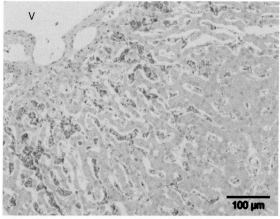

Figure 4.18 Dog. Chronic passive congestion. Perivenous fibrosis with dilated lymphatics, centrolobular atrophy of the hepatic cords and hepatocellular regeneration as evidenced by double layered hepatic cords in the periportal parenchyma (lower right). HE. V – hepatic vein.

perivenular fibrosis (Fig. 4.18) and deposition of extracellular matrix in the walls of the affected sinusoids, eventually leading to bridging fibrosis linking hepatic venules, and finally so called cardiac cirrhosis. In chronic passive congestion, hepatocellular regeneration as a consequence of loss of functional hepatic parenchyma, will often be evident in the presence of double layered hepatic cords in the unaffected periportal areas (Fig. 4.18). In acute or recurrent severe disruptions of the hepatic outflow, ischemic hepatic necrosis is regularly observed (Fig. 4.19). Passive congestion also causes

increased lymph production and dilated lymphatics are seen in the Glisson's capsule, the portal areas and around the larger hepatic veins.

Macroscopically the liver becomes swollen, dark and congested, often with an accentuated lobular pattern (nutmeg appearance) caused by centrilobular congestion contrasting with periportal steatosis or hyperplasia of hepatocytes (Fig. 4.20). The increased venous pressure may also lead to transudation of plasma and erythrocytes through the

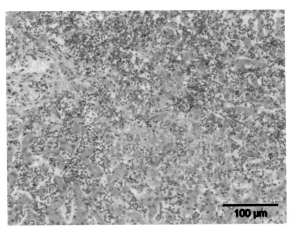

Figure 4.19 Dog. Passive congestion and ischemic hepatocellular necrosis. HE.

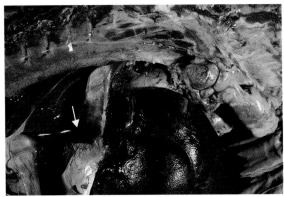

Figure 4.21 Dog. Passive congestion of the liver (swollen, dark, fibrin on the surface) due to expansion of an adrenocortical tumour (A) along the posterior caval vein up to the thoracic segment (arrow). (Reproduced from van den Ingh TS, Rothuizen J, Meyer HP. Circulatory disorders of the liver in dogs and cats. Vet Q 1995; 17(2):70–76, with permission)

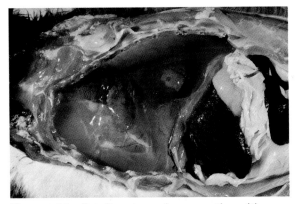

Figure 4.20 Cat. Chronic passive congestion with an accentuated lobular pattern due to centrolobular congestion and periportal hepatocellular regeneration. Cardiac pulmonary stenosis.

capsule. As a result, fibrin plaques may develop on the surface of the liver (Fig. 4.21) and blood-tinged fluid may accumulate in the abdominal cavity. In chronic stages the capsule becomes thickened by fibrosis as a result of the organization of the fibrin plaques.

In dogs and cats, passive congestion of the liver is usually the consequence of **cardiac failure** as in congenital cardiac anomalies (Fig. 4.18), valvular endocarditis or endocardiosis, myocardial damage, and pericardial effusion. Passive congestion may also result from partial or complete **obstruction**

(e.g. thrombosis, neoplasia, dirofilariasis) **or compression** (a.o. neoplasia, inflammation) **of the caudal caval vein** downstream from or at the outflow site of the hepatic veins (Fig. 4.21). Passive congestion due to **intrahepatic outflow disturbances** is associated with obstruction of the hepatic veins. Thrombotic obstruction of the larger hepatic veins, as in human Budd Chiari syndrome has not been conclusively reported in dogs and cats. Canine and feline cases reported as Budd Chiari-like syndrome,[15–19] terminology that we consider to be misleading and that we can do without, were associated with passive congestion caused by obstruction or compression of the caudal caval vein or perivenular fibrosis of the intrahepatic veins. Veno-occlusive disease, i.e. occlusion of terminal and intercalated (sublobular) hepatic veins by intimal thickening with loosely arranged or dense fibrous connective tissue, occurs in humans and animals (Fig. 4.22). This syndrome is associated with ingestion of pyrrolizidine alkaloids and, in humankind, with anticancer therapy such as irradiation and chemotherapy. Veno-occlusive disease does not occur spontaneously in dogs or cats, but it has been produced experimentally in dogs[20] and occurs spontaneously in wild felidae (cheetah and snow leopard).[21,22]

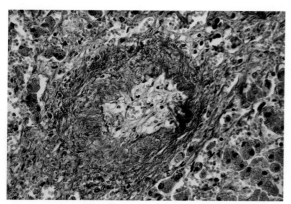

Figure 4.22   Cheetah. Veno-occlusive disease (Von Gieson – Elastica stain).

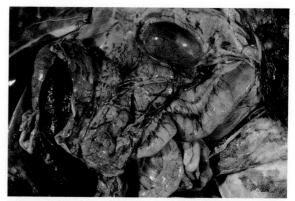

Figure 4.23   Dog. Multiple portosystemic collaterals: spleno-renal and mesenteric anastomoses secondary to portal hypertension. (Reproduced from van den Ingh TS, Rothuizen J, Meyer HP. Circulatory disorders of the liver in dogs and cats. Vet Q 1995; 17(2):70–76, with permission).

Disorders associated with portal hypertension

Portal hypertension is the abnormal state of a persistent increase in pressure in the portal venous system. Consequently, it is often accompanied by ascites and acquired portosystemic shunting via collateral vessels. In contrast to humankind, congestive splenomegaly is not a feature of portal hypertension in dogs and cats. In the normal dog and cat, these portosystemic collaterals are small and insignificant, but dilatation develops in response to portal hypertension, so that the high pressure is relieved by the patent connection of the portal system with the systemic venous circulation, in which the pressure is normally low. These vessels only become functional if there is a pressure gradient between the portal and systemic circulation, hence not in the case of generalized hypertension. Functional collaterals become visible as multiple, tortuous vessels particularly in the mediastinum along the esophagus originating from the cardia of the stomach (cardioesophageal anastomoses), in the omentum between the spleen and the left dorsal abdominal wall cranial to the kidney (spleno-renal anastomoses), and in the mesocolon and mesorectum (mesenteric anastomoses).[23,24] Portal hypertension with portosystemic collaterals is regularly seen in dogs (Fig. 4.23) but rare in cats (Fig. 4.24). It may result from primary vascular disorders or primary hepatic diseases. Portal hypertension may also occur in passive congestion of the liver but then it is not associated with acquired por-

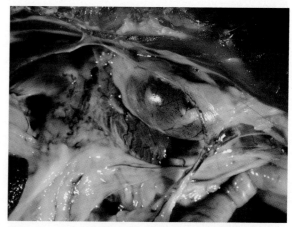

Figure 4.24   Cat. Multiple portosystemic collaterals: spleno-renal and mesenteric anastomoses secondary to portal hypertension.

tosystemic collaterals due to the absence of a pressure gradient.

Primary vascular disorders

Portal vein obstruction   Portal vein obstruction can occur from intraluminal disorders, such as thrombosis (Fig. 4.25) induced by damage to the portal vein by local inflammatory processes as in pancreatitis, ascending omphalophlebitis, and focal

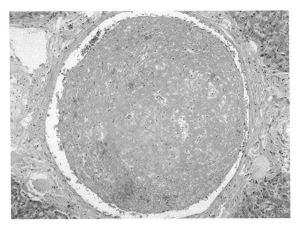

Figure 4.25   Dog. Thrombosis of the portal vein. HE.

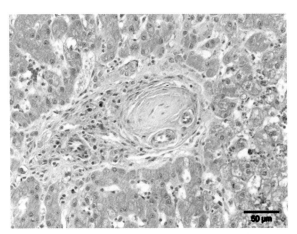

Figure 4.26   Dog. Obliteration due to fibrosis of the portal vein and arteriolar proliferation. HE.

or diffuse peritonitis, or by hypercoagulable states.[9,25] Neoplasia may occasionally cause obstruction of the portal vein by direct invasion and expansion in the portal vein or by embolization of portal veins. Circumscribed fibrosis of the wall and constriction of the extrahepatic portal vein[26] or compression of the extrahepatic portal vein due to local inflammatory lesions, such as abscesses or local neoplasms, can also occur and reduce or completely arrest portal blood flow. Histologically, the intrahepatic portal veins may be reduced in size depending on the degree and duration of reduced portal vein flow and this change may occur along with an increase in the number of arteriolar profiles in the portal tracts (Fig. 4.26). These changes are not specific for portal vein obstruction and additional clinical, biochemical or imaging information may be needed to make a diagnosis. In some circumstances etiologic clues may be present in the liver biopsy such as disseminated tumor emboli or a multifocal distribution of inflammatory foci or thrombi depending on the cause of the portal vein obstruction. These features may help to distinguish portal vein obstruction from other causes of reduced portal vein flow.

A special form of portal vein obstruction and possible subsequent portal hypertension is seen in dogs after parasitic infestation with trematodes of the genus *Schistosoma japonicum* (East Asia) and *Heterobilharzia americana* (North America).[27,28] The adult worms live in the mesenteric veins; their ova, which circulate as emboli can lodge in the smaller intrahepatic portal vein branches and, as foreign bodies, cause chronic granulomatous inflammation in the portal veins and surrounding portal areas.

Primary hypoplasia of the portal vein   Primary hypoplasia of the portal vein is a congenital disorder which occurs in dogs and very seldom in cats.[9,29] Several diagnostic terms have been used until now to identify this congenital condition (non-cirrhotic portal hypertension,[30] hepatoportal fibrosis[31]), but our preference is primary hypoplasia of the portal vein. Microvascular dysplasia,[32–34] as reported in dogs, shows the stereotypical histological picture of portal vein hypoperfusion. In the available literature there have been no clinical or biochemical findings to suggest that this disease (mild forms of) is different from primary portal vein hypoplasia. The authors involved in this standardization effort have therefore decided to abandon the name microvascular dysplasia, since the disease had already been reported before as primary portal vein hypoplasia, which gives a better description of the disease.

The disorder has a wide variation in clinical severity and morphology depending on the degree of hypoplasia of the portal vein and consequent acquired portosystemic collateral circulation and loss of hepatocellular function. The hypoplasia most likely affects both the extrahepatic (Fig. 4.27) and the intrahepatic segments of the portal vein. However, due to lack of objective criteria,

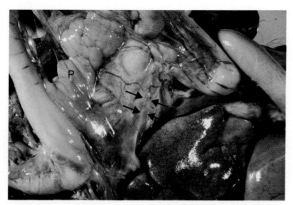

Figure 4.27 Dog. Primary hypoplasia of the portal vein. Marked gross hypoplasia of the extrahepatic portal vein (arrows). C – posterior caval vein. P – pancreas. (Reproduced from van den Ingh TS, Rothuizen J, Meyer HP. Portal hypertension associated with primary hypoplasia of the hepatic portal vein in dogs. Vet Rec 1995; 137(17):424–427, with permission)

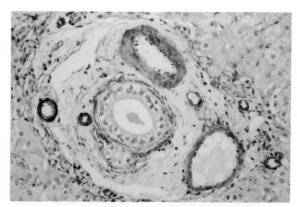

Figure 4.28 Dog. Primary hypoplasia of the portal vein. Decreased diameter of the portal vein and slight arteriolar proliferation. Immunohistochemical stain for alpha-smooth muscle actin.

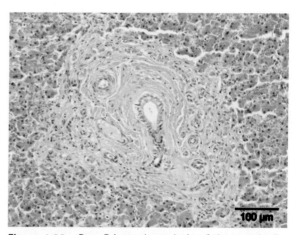

Figure 4.29 Dog. Primary hypoplasia of the portal vein. Portal fibrosis, no recognizable portal vein, arteriolar and bile duct proliferation. HE.

hypoplasia of the extrahepatic portal vein may easily be overlooked. Histologically, the disorder shares many histological features with other diseases causing hypoperfusion of the portal vein such as congenital portosystemic shunts, intrahepatic arterioportal fistulas (vide infra) and portal vein obstruction. Typically there is a decreased portal vein diameter or absence of the portal vein and an increased number of arteriolar profiles in the portal tracts. In about 30% of dogs with primary hypoplasia of the portal vein the vascular changes are mild and there is no evidence of portal fibrosis (Fig. 4.28); the other cases are characterized by moderate to marked fibrosis of the portal tracts sometimes resulting in portoportal fibrosis, hypoplasia or absence of the portal veins, and a varying proliferation of arterioles and bile ductules, particularly at the periphery of the portal areas (Fig. 4.29).[29] Hepatocytes are usually atrophic and lobules are small. Lymphatics may be distended. Clinical signs may become manifest between 1 month and 4 years of age and result from portal hypertension with development of multiple portosystemic collaterals and secondary hepatic atrophy. Some animals have ascites and hepatoencephalopathy at presentation while others may develop these signs later in the course of their disease depending on the degree of abnormality in the portal vasculature. The diagnosis is based on

histological examination of a liver biopsy in combination with ultrasonographic findings which exclude the presence of a congenital portosystemic shunt, an arteriovenous fistula, or portal vein thrombosis. In mild cases there are no ultasonographic changes at all. In more severe cases there may be portal hypertension, retrograde portal flow, ascites and multiple portosystemic collaterals.

Intrahepatic arterio-venous fistulas Intrahepatic arterio-venous fistulas occur in young dogs and cats.[35,36] In both species the disorder is presumed to be a congenital abnormality and represents communications between the hepatic artery and portal

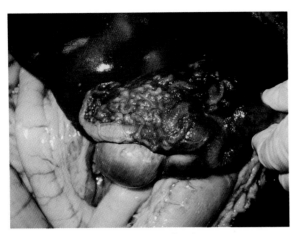

Figure 4.30   Dog. Arterioportal fistula.

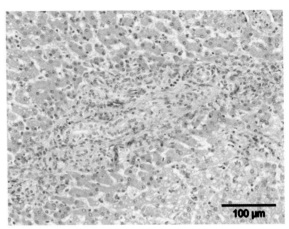

Figure 4.32   Dog. Arterioportal fistula. Portal area aside of the primary lesion with hypoplasia of the portal vein and marked arteriolar proliferation. HE.

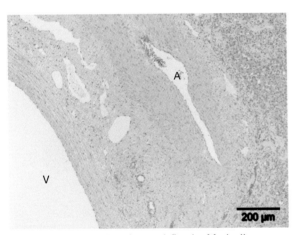

Figure 4.31   Dog. Arterioportal fistula. Markedly distended portal vein (V) with smooth muscle hypertrophy, hypertrophic hepatic artery (A) and fibrosis of the remaining liver tissue (upper right). HE.

venous radicles with subsequent retrograde flow in the portal vein and portal hypertension. One or more lobes may be affected, which usually reveal aneurysmal distension of pulsating portal veins and are supplied by one or several thick walled tortuous hepatic arteries (Fig. 4.30). Histologically, the affected lobes show distended portal veins with damaged walls characterized by intimal and medial fibroelastosis and smooth muscle hypertrophy, multiple cross sections of hypertrophic hepatic arteries and often atrophy and fibrosis of the adjacent hepatic tissue (Fig. 4.31). Sometimes second-

ary portal vein thrombosis and reorganisation may be seen. Portal tracts aside of the primary lesion in the affected lobe(s) and in the non-affected lobes often show hypoplasia of the portal vein with an increased number of arteriolar and sometimes also ductular profiles (Fig. 4.32). If the fistula is missed at clinical examination or surgery the histology of this disorder is difficult to distinguish from congenital portosystemic shunts and primary hypoplasia of the portal vein, since the histological appearance of the portal tracts in the non-affected lobes are similar. We have the strong impression that in dogs, arteriovenous fistulas are very often associated with the primary form of portal vein hypoplasia. One argument for this is that recovery of portal vein hypoplasia has never been recorded after surgical correction of the fistula by resection of the affected lobe. Arteriovenous shunts in extrahepatic splanchnic or umbilical (authors' observations) location may also produce portal hypertension.

Primary hepatic disease

Portal hypertension in the dog is usually the result of advanced chronic liver disease such as macronodular and micronodular cirrhosis, lobular dissecting hepatitis and very chronic extrahepatic cholestasis (biliary fibrosis). Portal hypertension in such cases is attributed to compression of the

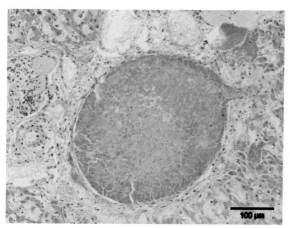

Figure 4.33 Kitten. Septic thrombosis of the portal vein with many bacteria. Fibrinous deposition, dilated lymphatics and many bacteria in the surrounding tissue. HE.

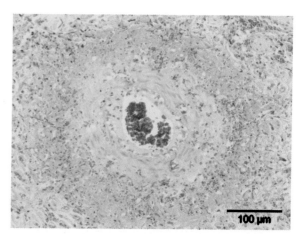

Figure 4.34 Dog. Fibrinoid periarteritis hepatic artery. HE.

portal and hepatic veins, increased resistance to sinusoidal blood flow, the formation of arteriovenous anastomoses particularly in the fibrous septa of cirrhotic livers, and increased portal flow (hyperdynamic portal circulation). In the cat, portal hypertension is particularly associated with chronic biliary inflammatory disease associated with marked biliary fibrosis. Also, in both species, congenital cystic disease of the liver with advanced portal fibrosis may result in portal hypertension.

OTHER VASCULAR DISORDERS

Thrombophlebitis of the portal vein and its tributaries can occur as mentioned above in ascending omphalophlebitis (Fig. 4.33), or in association with focal or diffuse inflammatory processes in the abdominal cavity (pancreas, spleen, stomach, intestine, peritoneum). The main consequence may be obstruction of the portal vein (vide supra) or extension of the inflammation from the affected portal vein branches into the connective tissue of the portal area or into the liver parenchyma to produce suppurative, necrotizing or granulomatous inflammation.

The hepatic artery is susceptible to diseases found in other arteries: arteriosclerosis and atherosclerosis, periarteritis nodosa and amyloidosis. The histological appearance is identical to that seen in other tissues, but it is rarely of clinical signifi-

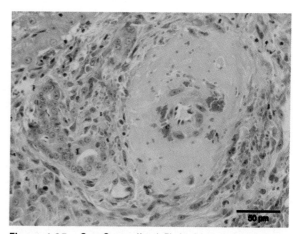

Figure 4.35 Cat. Generalized fibrinoid periarteritis with some reactive fibrosis and biliary proliferation. HE.

cance. Particularly in **periarteritis nodosa** (Figs 4.34, 4.35), inflammation or the secondary ischemia may affect other structures in the portal tracts or even cause parenchymal necrotic lesions.

DIAGNOSTIC METHODS REQUIRED FOR DIAGNOSIS OF CIRCULATORY DISORDERS OF THE LIVER

Vascular liver diseases are often accompanied by portosystemic collateral circulation. In the case of congenital portosystemic shunts (CPSSs) this causes almost complete shunting of portal blood past the liver, and poor growth and development of the liver which falls behind as the animal grows. This discrepancy causes clinical signs usually starting around 6 months of age. Also in other congenital diseases of the portal vein, such as primary portal vein hypoplasia and arteriovenous fistulas the liver is poorly perfused and does not grow adequately. Portal hypertension often leads to acquired collateral shunting of portal blood, and these animals also present symptoms of portosystemic shunting and have a small liver. However, circulatory diseases acquired later in life, such as portal vein thrombosis or chronic hepatitis, also lead to a decreased liver mass and portal hypertension. Depending on how severe and prolonged portal hypertension is, these diseases may also cause acquired portosystemic collateral circulation, and again, symptoms related to a too small liver. Diseases such as primary portal vein hypoplasia and chronic hepatitis may vary much in their severity and hence clinical presentation. The liver may be very small or normal in size and portal hypertension and acquired formation of portosystemic collaterals may be pronounced or slight to absent. The principle difference between congenital portosystemic shunts and the other circulatory liver diseases is that animals with CPSS never have portal hypertension, and therefore do not display ascites. The other primary or acquired circulatory diseases are associated with portal hypertension which may, if severe enough, cause ascites.

Tests to demonstrate (or exclude) portosystemic shunting

Portosystemic shunting may be congenital or acquired. In congenital portosystemic shunts, nearly all portal blood bypasses the liver; in porta-(hemi)azygos shunts the shunting fraction may be lower because the receiving vessel is relatively small and presents resistance to the shunting blood. The symptoms of hepatic encephalopathy, vomiting and polydipsia/polyuria which are classic for all forms of portosystemic shunting may be less pronounced or nearly absent in dogs with porta-(hemi)azygos shunts. Dogs with porta-azygos shunts may become symptomatic when they are much older than dogs with porta-cava shunts. Dogs with

acquired shunts due to portal hypertension may present at any age, naturally depending on the underlying cause. Acquired portosystemic shunting may vary from slight to very pronounced, so that related symptoms and blood changes may also vary. Acquired portosystemic shunting is very rare in cats and is almost exclusively associated with very chronic lymphocytic cholangitis.

The classical blood tests to demonstrate portosystemic shunting are plasma bile acids with 1.5 hour postprandial bile acid levels as the related challenge test,[37] and plasma ammonia which may be extended to the rectal or oral ammonial tolerance test.[38,39] Bile acid concentrations are influenced by decreased clearance by the liver in case of portosystemic collateral circulation, but also by reflux of bile components to the bloodstream via the hepatic lymphatic system (cholestasis). Cholestasis occurs in nearly all parenchymal hepatic and biliary diseases so that bile acid concentrations (basal and post-prandrially) may be increased in many hepatobiliary diseases. Bile acid measurement is therefore less suitable to demonstrate portosystemic shunting in a clinical population that contains many patients with liver disease.

Plasma ammonia is much more specific to demonstrate portosystemic shunting, also in a population of patients with liver disease.[39] Apart from the extremely rare inborn errors of ammonia metabolism,[41] portosystemic shunting is the only way ammonia can be increased.[40] In the case of severe liver dysfunction without portosystemic shunting the reserve capacity of the liver is adequate enough to keep ammonia within reference limits and to prevent the ammonia tolerance test becoming abnormal. The only parenchymal disease which may cause hyperammonemia without portal hypertension is fulminant hepatitis. This disease may functionally be considered as a condition with extreme intrahepatic portosystemic shunting due to gross absence of liver parenchyma. The ammonia tolerance test is best tolerated when ammonia is given deep rectally (10–15 cm) via a catheter after a walk to empty the rectum. Oral administration may induce vomiting and requires restraint and administration via a gastric tube. The standard dose is 2 ml/kg of a 5% NH_4Cl solution, and blood sampling for ammonia measurement is done before and 20 and 40 min after administration. In case of portosystemic shunting there is at least a doubling of the basal level, but in nearly all cases with pronounced shunting (e.g. congenital portosystemic shunts) the challenged concentration is much higher. The short-lasting temporary increment of ammonia concentration during the ammonia tolerance test is never hazardous for the patient. Fasting ammonia concentrations exceeding 100 µmol/L (upper reference concentration is around 45 µmol/L) are diagnostic for portosystemic shunting and there is no indication for an ammonia tolerance test in such cases. The ammonia tolerance test is preferred over measurement of post-prandial ammonia, which is less distinct and predictable. Presently there are good and affordable ammonia analyzers for practice.[41] A blood sample for ammonia measurement should be processed immediately, or stored in melting ice until analysis, but never for longer than 40 min. Contact with ammonia contaminants such as saliva, sweat and cigarette smoke should be avoided. Hemolytic samples should not be processed because the concentration of ammonia is three times higher in the erythrocyte than in normal plasma.

Scintigraphic diagnosis of portosystemic shunting

Portosystemic shunting may be diagnosed by per rectal portal scintigraphy using ^{99m}Technetium pertechnetate.[42,43] In normal dogs, dynamic lateral scintigraphic images of the abdomen sequentially visualize the portal vein and liver, and several seconds later the heart and lungs. In the case of congenital portosystemic shunts the heart and lungs are visualized before the liver which receives most activity via the hepatic artery in the second circulation and not via the portal vein. Per rectal scintigraphy gives semi-quantitative information about the fraction of portal blood shunting past the liver. Precise measurement of the shunting fraction may be performed with another method of portal vein scintigraphy, in which suspended ^{99m}Tc-labeled albumin macroaggregate particles are injected in a splenic vein branch under ultrasound guidance.[44,45] The labelled particles are trapped in the first capillary bed encountered, which is normally the liver, but can be the lung in the case of

portosystemic shunting. The ratio (activity in lungs and liver):(activity in the liver) gives the shunting fraction.

The above-mentioned tests to confirm or exclude the presence of portosystemic shunting are usually not diagnostic for the underlying disease, but evaluate shunting irrespective of the cause. For the final diagnosis of a disease causing portosystemic shunting, a combination of different tests and criteria is necessary. Not all circulatory liver disorders are associated with portosystemic shunting (acquired or congenital) or portal hypertension.

PATHOPHYSIOLOGICAL CHANGES AND DIAGNOSTIC TESTS FOR CIRCULATORY LIVER DISEASES

A summary of pathophysiological changes and the value of diagnostic tests is given in Table 4.1.

SUMMARY

This chapter describes the nature and morphological characteristics of the normal hepatic circulation, consequences of impaired hepatic perfusion, the histological pattern of portal venous hypoperfusion, and the circulatory disorders of the liver in dogs and cats. Impaired hepatic perfusion can result in reduced portal flow, which leads to atrophy of (the deprived segment of) the liver, or ischemia and subsequent ischemic necrosis. Portal venous hypoperfusion causes a stereotypical histological response of the liver. In the portal tracts the profile of the portal vein becomes diminished or absent, the number of arteriolar profiles increases, and sometimes sinusoidal dilatation occurs in the periportal areas; fibrosis and an increased number of ductular profiles may also be present. Circulatory disorders of the liver can be grouped into three major categories: congenital portosystemic shunts, disorders with outflow disturbances resulting in passive congestion of the liver, and disorders associated with deranged inflow of portal blood and portal hypertension. Congenital portosystemic shunts (CPSSs) are single large caliber vascular anomalies that directly connect the portal venous system with the systemic venous circulation. The liver histologically shows the typical characteristics

Table 4.1 Summary of pathophysiologic characteristics of vascular diseases of the liver, and the role of different diagnostic tests

Disease	Portosystemic shunting		Portal hyper-tension	Ascites	Histology essential for diagnosis	Ultrasono-graphy essential for diagnosis
	Congenital, usually 90–100%	Acquired, all stages from mild to severe				
Congenital						
PS shunt	+	−	−	−	−[a]	+
Outflow disturbances	−	−	±	−/+	−	−/+
Portal vein obstruction	−	−/±/+	±/+	±/+	−[a]	+
Arteriovenous fistula	−	±/+	+	±/+	−[a]	+
Portal vein hypoplasia[b]	−	−/±/+	±/+	−/±/+	±	±
Primary hepatic diseases	−	−/±/+	−/±/+	−/±/+	+	±

− = not true; + = essential
[a]These diseases have identical histopathological changes
[b]No single test is diagnostic; combined results should be evaluated

of portal venous hypoperfusion. Outflow disturbances of the liver result in acute or chronic passive congestion and are usually the result of cardiac failure. Portal hypertension with resultant portosystemic collateral circulation and ascites mainly results from chronic primary liver disease, particularly cirrhosis. Portal hypertension may also be the result of primary vascular lesions, such as primary hypoplasia of the portal vein, obstruction (thrombosis) of the portal vein, and intrahepatic arterioportal fistula. Primary hypoplasia of the portal vein histologically shows the typical pattern of portal venous hypoperfusion. Animals with long-standing portal vein obstruction and intrahepatic arterioportal fistulas, apart from the usually localized primary lesion, often also show this pattern with hypoplasia of the portal vein and an increased number of arteriolar profiles in the portal tracts.

References

1. McSween RNM, Desmet VJ, Roskams T, et al. Developmental anatomy and normal structure. In: McSween RNM, Burt AD, Portmann BC, et al, eds. Pathology of the liver. 4th edn. London: Churchill Livingstone; 2002:3–66.
2. Wilkens H, Münster W. Eingeweidevenen der V.cava caudalis. In: Nickel R, Schummer A, Seiferle E, eds. Lehrbuch der Anatomie der Haustiere. Berlin: Paul Parey Verlag; 1976:268–273.
3. Kalt DJ, Stump JE. Gross anatomy of the canine portal vein. Anat Histol Embryol 1993; 22: 191–197.
4. Payne JT, Martin RA, Constantinescu GM. The anatomy and embryology of portosystemic shunts in dogs and cats. Semin Vet Med Surg (Small Anim) 1990; 5:76–82.
5. Yamamoto K. Ultrastructural study on the venous sphincter in the sublobular vein of the canine liver. Microvasc Res 1998; 55(3):215–222.
6. Hanson KM, Johnson PC. Local control of hepatic arterial and portal venous flow in the dog. Am J Physiol 1966; 211:712–720.
7. Campra JL, Reynolds TB. The hepatic circulation. In: Arias IM, Jakoby WB, Popper H, et al, eds. The liver: biology and pathobiology. 2nd edn. New York: Raven Press; 1988:911–930.
8. Lohse CL, Suter PF. Functional closure of the ductus venosus during early postnatal life in the dog. Am J Vet Res 1977; 38:839–844.
9. van den Ingh TS, Rothuizen J, Meyer HP. Circulatory disorders of the liver in dogs and cats. Vet Q 1995; 17(2):70–76.
10. Inoue S, Matsunuma N, Ono K, et al. Five cases of canine peliosis hepatis. Nippon Juigaku Zasshi 1988; 50(2):565–567.
11. Brown PJ, Henderson JP, Galloway P, et al. Peliosis hepatis and teleangiectasis in 18 cats. J Small Anim Pract 1994; 35:73–77.

12. Cullen JM, MacLachlan NJ. Liver, biliary system and pancreas. In: McGavin MD, Carlton WW, Zachary JF, eds. Thomson's Special Veterinary Pathology. St. Louis; 2001:81–123.

13. Kelly WR. The liver and biliary system. In: Jubb KVF, Kennedy PC, Palmer N, eds. Pathology of domestic animals. 4th edn. San Diego: Academic Press; 1992: 319–406.

14. Wanless IR. Vascular disorders. In: McSween RNM, Burt AD, Portmann BC, eds. Pathology of the liver. 4th edn. London: Churchill Livingstone; 2002: 539–573.

15. Cohn LA, Spaulding KA, Cullen JM, et al. Intrahepatic postsinusoidal venous obstruction in a dog. J Vet Intern Med 1991; 5(6):317–321.

16. MacIntire DK, Henderson RH, Banfield C, et al. Budd-Chiari syndrome in a kitten, caused by membranous obstruction of the caudal vena cava. J Am Anim Hosp Assoc 1995; 31(6):484–491.

17. Fine DM, Olivier NB, Walshaw R, et al. Surgical correction of late-onset Budd-Chiari-like syndrome in a dog. J Am Vet Med Assoc 1998; 212(6):835–837.

18. Schoeman JP, Stidworthy MF. Budd-Chiari-like syndrome associated with an adrenal phaeochromocytoma in a dog. J Small Anim Pract 2001; 42(4):191-194.

19. Cave TA, Martineau H, Dickie A, et al. Idiopathic hepatic veno-occlusive disease causing Budd-Chiari-like syndrome in a cat. J Small Anim Pract 2002; 43(9):411-415.

20. Schulman KB, Luk K, Deeg HJ, et al. Induction of hepatic veno-occlusive disease in dogs. Am J Pathol 1987; 126:114–125.

21. Gosselin SJ, Loudy DL, Tarr MJ, et al. Veno-occlusive disease of the liver in captive cheetah. Vet Pathol 1988; 25(1):48–57.

22. van den Ingh TS, Zwart P, Heldstab A. Veno-occlusive disease (VOD) of the liver in cheetahs and snowleopards. Schweiz Arch Tierheilkd 1981; 123(6):323–327.

23. Khan IR, Vitums A. Portosystemic communications in the cat. Res Vet Sci 1971; 12:215–218.

24. Vitums A. Portosystemic communications in the dog. Acta Anat 1959; 39:271–299.

25. van Winkle TJ, Bruce E. Thrombosis of the portal vein in eleven dogs. Vet Pathol 1993; 30:28–35.

26. Szatmari V, van den Ingh TS, Fenyves B, et al. Portal hypertension in a dog due to circumscribed fibrosis of the wall of the extrahepatic portal vein. Vet Rec 2002; 150(19):602–605.

27. Smith HA, Jones TC. Veterinary Pathology. 3rd edn. Philadelphia: Lea and Febiger; 1966.

28. Flowers JR, Hammerberg B, Wood SL, et al. Heterobilharzia americana infection in a dog. J Am Vet Med Assoc 2002; 220:193–196.

29. van den Ingh TS, Rothuizen J, Meyer HP. Portal hypertension associated with primary hypoplasia of the hepatic portal vein in dogs. Vet Rec 1995; 137(17):424–427.

30. Bunch SE, Johnson SE, Cullen JM. Idiopathic noncirrhotic portal hypertension in dogs: 33 cases (1982–1998). J Am Vet Med Assoc 2001; 218(3):392–399.

31. van Den Ingh TS, Rothuizen J. Hepatoportal fibrosis in three young dogs. Vet Rec 1982; 110(25):575–577.

32. Schermerhorn T, Center SA, Dykes NL, et al. Characterization of hepatoportal microvascular dysplasia in a kindred of cairn terriers. J Vet Intern Med 1996; 10:219–230.

33. Christiansen JS, Hottinger HA, Allen L, et al. Hepatic microvascular dysplasia in dogs: a retrospective study of 24 cases. J Am Anim Hosp Assoc 2000; 36:385–389.

34. Allen L, Stobie D, Mauldin GN, et al. Clinicopathologic features of dogs with hepatic microvascular dysplasia with and without portosystemic shunts: 42 cases (1991–1996). J Am Vet Med Assoc 1999; 214(2):218–220.

35. Moore PF, Whiting PG. Hepatic lesions associated with intrahepatic arterioportal fistulae in dogs. Vet Pathol 1986; 23(1):57–62.

36. Legendre AM, Krahwinkel DJ, Carrig CB, et al. Ascites associated with intrahepatic arteriovenous fistula in a cat. J Am Vet Med Assoc 1976; 168:589–591.

37. Kerr MG, van Doorn T. Mass screening of Irish wolfhound puppies for portosystemic shunts by the dynamic bile acid test. Vet Rec 1999; 144(25):693–696.

38. Rothuizen J, van den Ingh TS. Rectal ammonia tolerance test in the evaluation of portal circulation in dogs with liver disease. Res Vet Sci 1982; 33(1):22–25.

39. Rothuizen J, van den Ingh TS. Arterial and venous ammonia concentrations in the diagnosis of canine hepato-encephalopathy. Res Vet Sci 1982; 33(1):17–21.

40. Meyer HP, Rothuizen J, Tiemessen I, et al. Transient metabolic hyperammonaemia in young Irish wolfhounds. Vet Rec 1996; 138(5): 105–107.

41. Sterczer A, Meyer HP, Boswijk HC, et al. Evaluation of ammonia measurements in dogs with two analysers

for use in veterinary practice. Vet Rec 1999; 144(19):523–526.

42. Daniel GB, Bright R, Ollis P, et al. Per rectal portal scintigraphy using 99mtechnetium pertechnetate to diagnose portosystemic shunts in dogs and cats. J Vet Intern Med 1991; 5(1):23–27.

43. Koblik PD, Komtebedde J, Yen CK, et al. Use of transcolonic 99mtechnetium-pertechnetate as a screening test for portosystemic shunts in dogs. J Am Vet Med Assoc 1990; 196(6):925–930.

44. Meyer HP, Rothuizen J, van den Brom WE, et al. Quantitation of portosystemic shunting in dogs by ultrasound-guided injection of 99MTc-macroaggregates into a splenic vein. Res Vet Sci 1994; 57(1):58–62.

45. Meyer HP, Rothuizen J, van Sluijs FJ, et al. Progressive remission of portosystemic shunting in 23 dogs after partial closure of congenital portosystemic shunts. Vet Rec 1999; 144(13):333–337.

Chapter 5

Morphological classification of biliary disorders of the canine and feline liver

Ted S. G. A. M van den Ingh, John M. Cullen, David C. Twedt, Tom Van Winkle, Valeer J. Desmet, Jan Rothuizen

CHAPTER CONTENTS

INTRODUCTION

The anatomy of the biliary system and the classification and morphology of the various biliary disorders in dogs and cats is presented in this chapter. The biliary disorders can be grouped into four major categories:

1. Biliary cystic disease and biliary atresia
2. Cholestasis and cholatestasis
3. Cholangitis
4. Diseases of the gall bladder.

Histological examination of liver biopsies can substantially aid in the diagnosis of the first three categories. Changes in the portal tracts are the hallmarks of most of these biliary disorders. However, portal inflammation, fibrosis and bile duct proliferation are not restricted to biliary disorders and may also be seen in primary parenchymal disorders such as acute and chronic hepatitis, and primary vascular abnormalities. Differentiation in general is possible through careful histological examination and evaluation of the combination of the parenchymal, vascular and portal tract lesions present in the affected liver. In contrast to parenchymal and neoplastic liver diseases the diagnosis of diseases of the biliary tract depends not only on histopathological evaluation, but also largely on ultrasonography. In neutrophilic cholangitis and cholecystitis culture and cytological examination of bile are required to assess the diagnosis.

The role of the different diagnostic methods is summarized at the end of the chapter.

ANATOMY OF THE BILIARY SYSTEM

The liver can be regarded as an exocrine gland and the smallest structures, the bile canaliculi, consist of intercellular spaces formed by the secretory hepatocytes that are sealed off by tight junctions between adjacent hepatocytes. The bile canalicular membrane represents a specialized area of the liver cell surface as evidenced, e.g. by the high concentration of alkaline phosphatase and the presence of a contractile actin filament network in the pericanalicular cytoplasma. In the periportal areas the bile canaliculi drain into cholangioles or terminal ductules (also known as canals of Hering), which are lined by ductal cells and hepatocytes. The ductules extend through the limiting plate and within the smallest portal tracts unite to form the interlobular bile ducts which are lined with cuboidal epithelium. The interlobular ducts anastomose and form the larger intrahepatic bile ducts lined with tall columnar epithelium with a basally located nucleus. These finally enter the main hepatic ducts that unite to form the common bile duct (also known as 'ductus choledochus') which enters the duodenum at the Vater's papilla. The gall bladder, responsible for storage and concentration of bile, communicates with the main hepatic ducts and the common bile duct via the cystic duct.[1-5]

BILIARY CYSTIC DISEASE AND BILIARY ATRESIA

Solitary cysts

Solitary cysts are rarely observed in dogs and cats (Fig. 5.1). They may vary markedly in size and are lined by a single layer of biliary epithelium (Fig. 5.2). They may be acquired or may be part of congenital cystic disease of the liver.

Congenital cystic disease of the liver

Congenital cystic disease of the liver is a complex and difficult group of diseases, which has caused much confusion in veterinary literature with respect to nomenclature and classification of the various disease entities. The proposed nomencla-

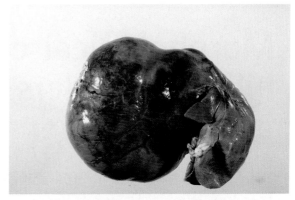

Figure 5.1   Cat. Solitary cyst. Formalin fixed specimen.

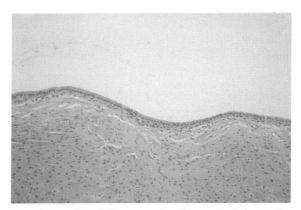

Figure 5.2   Cat. Solitary cyst lined by a single layer of epithelium. HE.

ture and classification of congenital cystic diseases in dogs and cats therefore is only understandable with knowledge of the embryological development of the biliary tree and the most recent human classification.

The various congenital cystic diseases of the liver, although quite different in appearance, are thought to represent anomalous development of the intrahepatic bile ducts, i.e. ductal plate anomalies, at different levels of the biliary tree.[6,7] In early gestation the liver develops from the hepatic diverticulum of the foregut, which comprises two parts: a cranial or hepatic part and a caudal or cystic part. The hepatic part gives rise to primitive liver cells growing into the vascularized mesenchyme of the septum transversum and thus forming a plate of liver cells alternating with hepatic sinusoids. The cystic part gives rise to the gall bladder and the common bile duct. In early development the liver has no intrahepatic bile duct system and hepatic artery, only primitive portal areas consisting of a portal vein surrounded by a myofibroblast-rich stroma. The bile ducts develop from a ring of primitive liver cells surrounding the primitive stroma around the portal veins, called the ductal plate, by regional duplication with subsequent focal dilatation and tubular formation and finally incorporation as individual bile ducts in the stromal tissue of the primitive portal area.[1,7–9] The development of the hepatic artery, most likely by vasogenesis from myofibroblasts in the primitive portal areas, precedes the incorporation of the tubular part of the ductal plate into the primitive portal area, and is essential for this incorporation.[10] As the formation of the intrahepatic bile ducts follows the outgrowth and development of the portal vein branches, the process results in a continuous development of bile ducts throughout fetal life from the liver hilus to the periphery.[1,7–9]

Congenital cystic diseases of the liver are characterized by dilatation of segments of the intrahepatic bile ducts and variable degrees of fibrosis, and are frequently associated with polycystic kidney disease. Although the hepatic lesions may show overlapping features, in humankind they can be classified according to their morphology and inheritance in three basic categories:

1. Autosomal recessive polycystic kidney disease (ARPKD) or *childhood type of polycystic disease*
2. Autosomal dominant polycystic kidney disease (ADPKD) or *adult type polycystic disease*
3. *Caroli's disease* with autosomal recessive inheritance.

In ARPKD the liver involvement is primarily microscopic and characterized by fibrotic portal areas with abnormally structured, often dilated, small bile ducts; in the so-called juvenile type the fibrosis is much more extensive, which macroscopically may result in an enlarged and firm liver *(congenital hepatic fibrosis)*. In ADPKD the liver is grossly characterized by multiple unilocular or multilocular cysts ranging from less than 1 mm to more than 12 cm in diameter; they contain a clear, colorless fluid and microscopically, are lined by columnar or cuboidal epithelium; *Von Meyenburg complexes,* i.e. discrete fibrotic areas with small often irregularly formed bile ducts, are considered

as part of the spectrum of ADPKD. In Caroli's disease the lesion is characterized by macroscopically recognizable moniliform or saccular dilatations of the larger intrahepatic bile ducts, i.e. the hepatic ducts and the segmental ducts. Microscopically the cystic ducts are lined by cuboidal to tall columnar epithelium and the lumen may contain inspissated mucin and bile, and calcareous material. In ADPKD the kidneys are characterized by multiple rounded tubular cysts of varying size (mm to several cm), which may form in any segment of the nephron but involve only a small percentage of the nephron population. In ARPKD and Caroli's disease, identical renal lesions, also known as polycystic kidney type I, are seen and are characterized by diffuse involvement of the kidneys with dilatation of collecting ducts, thus producing a radial cystic pattern from papilla to cortical surface.[6,11,12]

The dilatation of the large intrahepatic bile ducts, as seen in Caroli's disease, is thought to represent an early defect in the formation of the intrahepatic bile ducts. The childhood type of polycystic disease including congenital hepatic fibrosis with abnormally structured cystic bile ducts therefore represents a ductal plate anomaly at an intermediate level. The unilocular and multilocular hepatic cysts and the Von Meyenburg complexes then represent a ductal plate anomaly at a late peripheral stage, whereby the large cysts may result from progressive dilatation of the Von Meyenburg complexes.[6,9]

Although often not clearly defined with regard to inheritance, similar morphological entities can be discriminated in dogs and cats. In these species we therefore propose to use the following terminologies for the hepatic lesions: **congenital dilatation of the large and segmental bile ducts,** morphologically identical to Caroli's disease (Figs 5.3, 5.4, 5.5), **juvenile polycystic disease/congenital hepatic fibrosis** (Figs 5.6, 5.7), and **adult polycystic disease** (Figs 5.8, 5.9), **including Von Meyenburg complexes** (Fig. 5.10).[13,14]

As in humankind, in Persian cats and Persian crossbreeds with polycystic kidney disease (Fig. 5.11), the phenotype of the hepatic lesions is not always consistent as the kidney lesions may be associated with both juvenile polycystic disease/congenital hepatic fibrosis or multiple uni- or multilocular cysts or even combinations of both lesions.[15]

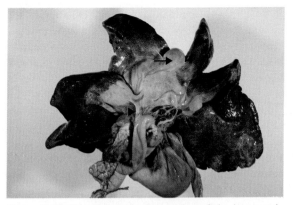

Figure 5.3   Dog. Congenital dilatation of the large and segmental bile ducts. The gall bladder (arrow) and the common bile duct (arrowhead) are normal in size. (Reproduced from Görlinger S, Rothuizen J, Bunch SE, et al. Congenital dilatation of the bile ducts (Caroli's disease) in young dogs. J Vet Intern Med 2003; 17:28–32, with permission).

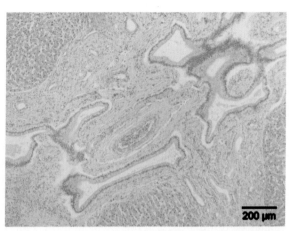

Figure 5.5   Dog. Congenital dilatation of the large and segmental bile ducts. Fibrotic portal area with dilated irregularly formed bile ducts lined with cylindrical epithelium. HE.

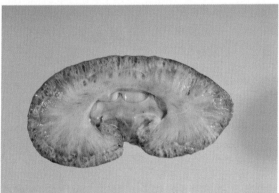

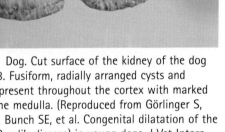

Figure 5.4   Dog. Cut surface of the kidney of the dog in Figure 5.3. Fusiform, radially arranged cysts and fibrosis are present throughout the cortex with marked fibrosis of the medulla. (Reproduced from Görlinger S, Rothuizen J, Bunch SE, et al. Congenital dilatation of the bile ducts (Caroli's disease) in young dogs. J Vet Intern Med 2003; 17:28–32, with permission).

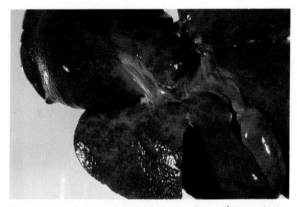

Figure 5.6   Cat. Juvenile polycystic disease/congenital hepatic fibrosis.

Biliary atresia

Biliary atresia is a very rare congenital anomaly in domestic animals and has been described only once in a dog.[16] The lesion was characterized by atresia of the common bile duct at the transition between the common bile duct and the hepatic ducts (Fig. 5.12) suggesting non-fusion of the cranial or hepatic and the caudal or cystic Anlage of the bile ducts. The animal was jaundiced from birth. At post-mortem examination there was complete absence of ductal structures at the site of the atresia. The liver showed histologically severe porto-portal bridging fibrosis with extensive biliary proliferation reminiscent of congenital hepatic fibrosis. This might indicate a combined anomalous development of extrahepatic and intrahepatic bile ducts in this dog, which corresponds with the occurrence of a ductal plate anomaly in 20–40% of human cases with extrahepatic biliary atresia.[17,18]

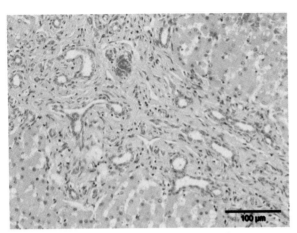

Figure 5.7   Cat. Juvenile polycystic disease/congenital hepatic fibrosis. Fibrotic portal area with irregularly formed slightly dilated bile ducts. HE.

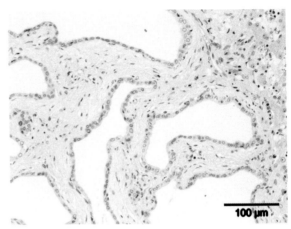

Figure 5.9   Cat. Adult polycystic disease. Fibrous tissue with irregularly formed cystic dilated bile ducts lined with a single layer of epithelium. HE.

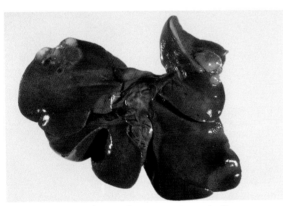

Figure 5.8   Cat (Persian). Adult polycystic disease. (Reproduced from Bosje JT, van den Ingh TS, van der Linde-Sipman JS. Polycystic kidney and liver disease in cats. Vet Q 1998; 20(4):136–139, with permission).

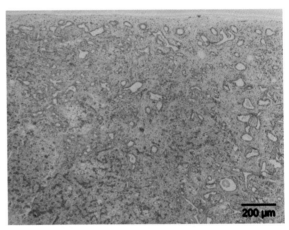

Figure 5.10   Dog. Von Meyenburg complex characterized by focal fibrosis and microscopically small, irregularly formed dilated bile ducts. HE.

CHOLESTASIS AND CHOLATE-STASIS

Cholestasis (bilirubinostasis)

Cholestasis (bilirubinostasis) is defined as impaired bile flow accompanied by the accumulation in the blood of components normally secreted in the bile (e.g. bile acids, conjugated bilirubin, cholesterol).[4] Morphologically, cholestasis (bilirubinostasis) is characterized by the presence of bile in the hepatic parenchyma and can be recognized as bile plugs in the canaliculi, phagocytosed bile (plugs) in Kupffer

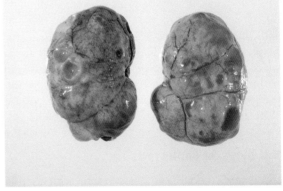

Figure 5.11   Cat. Polycystic kidney disease with multiple rounded cysts.

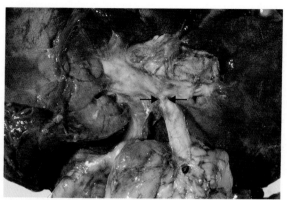

Figure 5.12 Dog. Extrahepatic biliary atresia. Atresia of the common bile duct (arrows) near the hilus of the liver. (Reproduced from Schulze C, Rothuizen J, van Sluijs FJ, et al. Extrahepatic biliary atresia in a border collie. J Small Anim Pract 2000; 41(1):27–30, with permission).

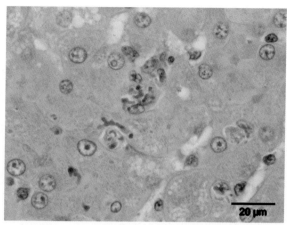

Figure 5.14 Dog. Bile plugs in the canaliculi and phagocytosed bile plugs in the Kupffer cells. HE.

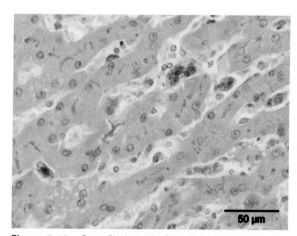

Figure 5.13 Dog. Cholestasis. Bile plugs in the canaliculi. HE.

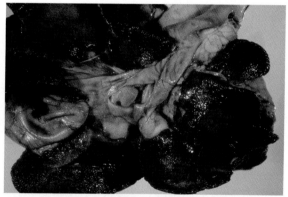

Figure 5.15 Dog. Extrahepatic cholestasis due to a gall stone with dilatation of the extrahepatic bile ducts.

cells/macrophages and as bile granules in the cytoplasm of hepatocytes (Figs 5.13, 5.14).[4] Cholestasis is easily recognized in cytological smears and frozen sections, but due to the paraffin embedding procedure, markedly less in paraffin sections of the same animals, particularly in cats.

Intrahepatic cholestasis

Intrahepatic cholestasis is associated with a wide spectrum of liver diseases. In general, microscopic lesions apart from the cholestasis are related to the

primary hepatic disease, but cholestasis may be the only histological abnormality.[19]

Extrahepatic cholestasis

Extrahepatic cholestasis can be associated with intraluminal obstruction (gall stones, mucinous cystic hyperplasia) or luminal constriction (neoplasia or inflammatory processes} of the extrahepatic biliary tract, and occasionally a large intrahepatic duct, and results in stasis of bile and dilatation of the bile ducts proximal to the obstruction (Fig. 5.15).

The characteristic microscopic lesions are related to the leakage of bile from the bile ducts into the

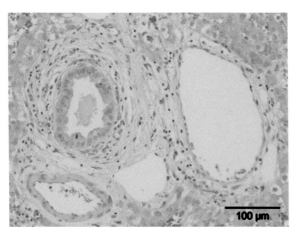

Figure 5.16   Dog. Acute extrahepatic cholestasis. Enlarged edematous portal area with a neutrophil portal infiltrate and slight proliferative reaction of the biliary epithelium. HE.

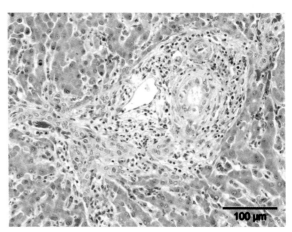

Figure 5.18   Dog. Chronic extrahepatic cholestasis with fibrosis, ductular proliferation and a mixed portal inflammatory infiltrate. HE.

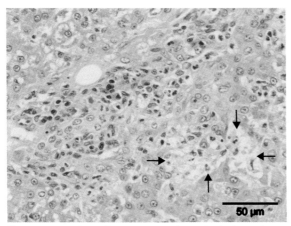

Figure 5.17   Dog. Subacute extrahepatic cholestasis with a mixed portal inflammatory infiltrate and slight ductular proliferation. A bile infarct is present in the periportal parenchyma (arrows). HE.

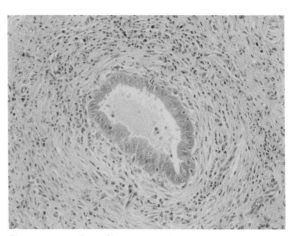

Figure 5.19   Dog. Chronic extrahepatic cholestasis with periductal concentric fibrosis and a mixed inflammatory infiltrate. HE.

connective tissue of the portal areas. In the **acute stage** this results in enlarged edematous portal tracts with a neutrophilic portal infiltrate and often, a degenerative and proliferative reaction of the bile duct epithelium (Fig. 5.16). Whereas cholestasis is a constant feature in acute extrahepatic cholestasis, bile infarcts, i.e. foci of hepatocellular necrosis due to insudation of extracellular bile (Fig. 5.17), although seen in other species, are mostly absent in dogs and cats. The **chronic stage** of extrahepatic cholestasis is characterized by enlarged portal areas with fibrosis, bile duct proliferation, periductal concentric fibrosis and an inflammatory infiltrate with pigment-laden macrophages, lymphocytes, plasma cells and neutrophils (Figs 5.18. 5.19). Histological evidence of cholestasis may be present or absent. In longstanding cases portoportal bridging fibrosis and eventually biliary fibrosis may develop.[19]

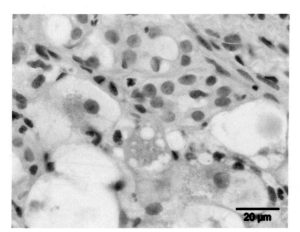

Figure 5.20 Dog. Cholate-stasis. Swollen, pale hepatocytes with centrally located copper-containing granules. HE.

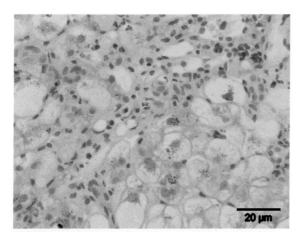

Figure 5.21 Dog. Cholatestasis. Swollen, pale hepatocytes with centrally located copper-containing granules. Rubeanic acid stain for copper.

Cholate-stasis

Cholate-stasis is a morphological entity well recognized in humankind and horses with chronic cholestatic liver diseases. The lesion is thought to be caused by the retention of bile acids in the hepatocytes, preferentially seen in the periportal region and often associated with ductular proliferation. The lesion is characterized by rounded swollen and pale hepatocytes with a distinct cell border and centrally located, often copper containing granules (Figs 5.20, 5.21).[4] It is a rare finding in dogs with chronic liver disease.

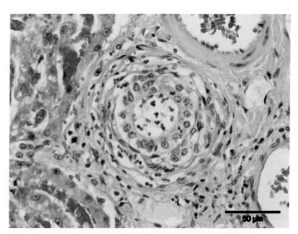

Figure 5.22 Cat. Neutrophilic cholangitis with extension of neutrophils in the portal area. HE.

CHOLANGITIS

Cholangitis can be split into four groups as follows:

1. neutrophilic cholangitis
2. lymphocytic cholangitis
3. destructive cholangitis
4. chronic cholangitis associated with liver fluke infestation.

Neutrophilic cholangitis

Neutrophilic cholangitis (also known as suppurative or exudative cholangitis/cholangiohepatitis) is the most common type of cholangitis, which is frequently seen in cats and rarely in dogs, and is believed to result from ascending bacterial infection from the intestine.[20–22] The lesion is histologically characterized by the presence of neutrophils in the lumen and/or epithelium of the bile ducts. In the acute stage the lesion is often associated with the presence of edema and neutrophils in the portal areas (Figs 5.22, 5.23). The neutrophilic inflammation may extend to the hepatic parenchyma and incidentally even result in hepatic abscesses. In the chronic stage the lesion is often associated with the presence of a mixed inflammatory infiltrate in the portal areas consisting of neutrophils, lymphocytes and plasma cells, and possibly fibrosis and bile ductular proliferation.

The lesions occur in varying intensity and may affect the liver diffusely as in severe disease or show

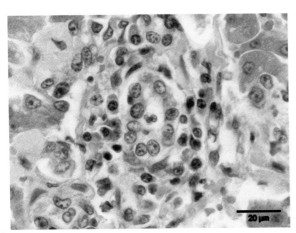

Figure 5.23 Cat. Neutrophilic cholangitis with a neutrophil in the lumen of the bile duct and some lymphocytes and plasma cells in the portal stromal tissue. HE.

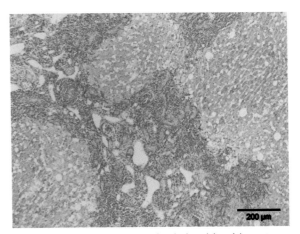

Figure 5.24 Cat. Lymphocytic cholangitis with porto-portal bridging. HE.

an irregular distribution with only limited numbers of portal tracts affected. Not all cases show the above typical changes; there may only be non-specific reactive hepatitis (Ch. 7).

Lymphocytic cholangitis

Lymphocytic cholangitis (also known as lympho-cytic cholangiohepatitis, lymphocytic portal hepa-titis, non-suppurative cholangitis)[20-23] is a rather common disease in cats with unknown etiology and pathogenesis. This is usually a very slowly pro-gressive and extremely chronic disease. The disease is characterized by a consistent infiltration of small lymphocytes in and restricted to the portal areas, often associated with variable portal fibrosis and biliary ductular proliferation (Figs 5.24, 5.25). Lymphocytes centering around the bile ducts or present in the biliary epithelium may be seen but are not a specific hallmark of the disease. Apart from lymphocytes, solitary plasma cells and eosinophils may be present. Note that well-differ-entiated lymphocytic malignant lymphoma may be difficult to discriminate from lymphocytic cholangitis.

Destructive cholangitis

Destructive cholangitis in dogs[24] is characterized by destruction and loss of the bile ducts in the

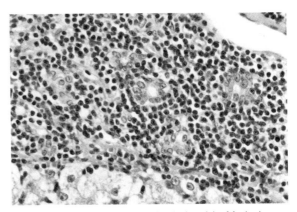

Figure 5.25 Cat. Lymphocytic cholangitis. Marked infiltration of small lymphocytes in the portal area and biliary proliferation. HE.

smaller portal areas with subsequent inflammation (pigment-laden macrophages, neutrophils and/or eosinophils) and eventually portal fibrosis (Fig. 5.26). It has been postulated that it results from an idiosyncratic reaction to drugs, particularly sulphonamides. However, viral infection, e.g. canine distemper (Fig. 5.27) and toxic insults may also be associated with the destruction of biliary epithelium. Destructive cholangitis usually causes very severe cholestasis and icterus. It is the only form of intrahepatic cholestasis that is so severe that acholic feces can be seen. This is otherwise a sign restricted to extrahepatic bile duct obstruc-tion. Whether or not destructive cholangitis results

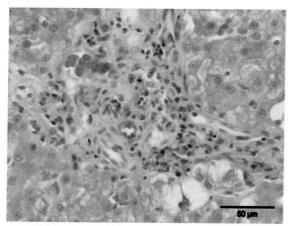

Figure 5.26 Dog. Destructive cholangitis. Idiosyncratic reaction to TMPS. HE.

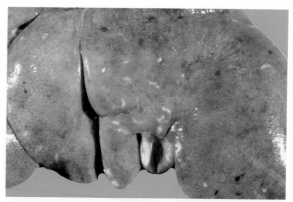

Figure 5.28 Cat. Chronic cholangitis due to liver fluke infestation.

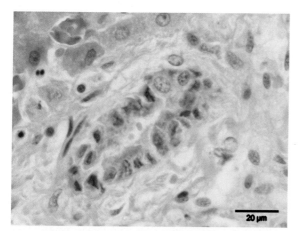

Figure 5.27 Dog. Destructive cholangitis with necrosis of the biliary epithelium and some intracytoplasmic viral inclusions. Canine distemper virus infection. HE.

Table 5.1 Species of Opisthorchiidae described in cats and dogs, and their geographic distribution (Reproduced from Bowman DD, Hendrix CM, Lindsay DS, et al. Feline clinical parasitology. 1st edn. Ames: Iowa State University Press; 2002, with permission of Blackwell Publishing)

Amphimerus pseudofelineus	North, Central and South America
Clonorchis sinensis	China, Japan, Korea, Taiwan
Opisthorchis felineus	Europe, Siberia, Ukraine
Opisthorchis viverrini	South Eastern Asia
Paropisthorchis caninus	India
Metorchis conjunctus	North America
Metorchis albidus	Northern Europe
Metorchis orientalis	South and Eastern Asia
Parametorchis complexum	USA
Pseudamphistomum truncatum	Europe, India

in definite destruction and loss of the bile ducts is unknown.

Chronic cholangitis associated with liver fluke infestation

Chronic cholangitis associated with liver fluke infestation is regularly observed in cats and less frequently in dogs in endemic areas. Infections are caused by members of the family Opisthorchiidae (Table 5.1), which require two intermediate hosts, the first being water snails and the second a wide variety of fish, in which the metacercariae are encysted. The final host acquires infection by inges-

tion of raw fish, and the young liver flukes migrate from the intestine to the liver via the bile ducts causing thickening and (cystic) dilatation of the ductus choledochus and large bile ducts (Fig. 5.28).[25,26] Microscopically, the lesion is characterized by dilated larger bile ducts with papillary projections and marked periductal and portal fibrosis (Figs 5.29, 5.30). A slight to moderate inflammation may be seen both within the ducts (neutrophils and macrophages) as well as in the portal areas (neutrophils, lymphocytes and plasma cells). Although eosinophils may be present, they are usually limited

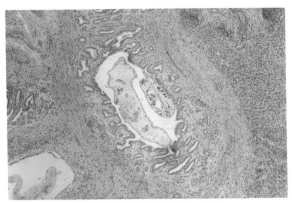

Figure 5.29   Cat. Chronic cholangitis due to liver fluke infestation with proliferation of the bile duct epithelium and marked periductal fibrosis. HE.

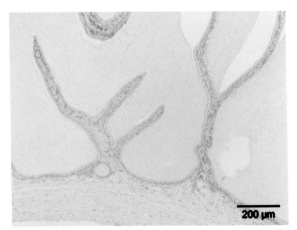

Figure 5.31   Dog. Cystic mucinous hyperplasia of the gallbladder. HE.

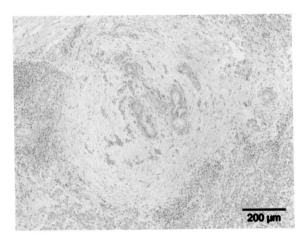

Figure 5.30   Cat. Chronic cholangitis due to liver fluke infestation with marked periductal fibrosis, biliary proliferation and peripherally located mononuclear inflammation. HE.

in numbers. The number of liver flukes and eggs within the dilated bile ducts varies markedly and generally, only limited evidence of liver flukes or eggs is seen.[25] In cats and dogs, chronic cholangitis due to liver fluke infestation has been associated with the development of intrahepatic and extrahepatic cholangiocellular carcinomas.[25]

DISEASES OF THE GALL BLADDER

Cystic mucinous hyperplasia

Cystic mucinous hyperplasia of the gall bladder is characterized by hyperplasia of the epithelium with

papillary projections and an increased mucin production (Fig. 5.31). With extreme mucin production the gall bladder may become markedly extended (**mucocele**) (Fig. 5.32) and may even rupture with or without preceding secondary neutrophilic cholecystitis.[27,28] In rare cases, the mucinous hyperplasia may include the extrahepatic bile ducts and cause extrahepatic cholestasis.[27] Gall bladder mucocele usually gives a typical ultrasonographic image of a dilated gallbladder with an orange-like radiated structure of the mucinous content (Fig. 5.33).

Cholecystitis

Neutrophilic cholecystitis is frequently seen in cats and rarely in dogs, and in general, is associated with bacterial infection. Neutrophilic cholecystitis can be present as a solitary lesion or in combination with neutrophilic cholangitis. The lesion is characterized by the presence of neutrophils in the lumen, the epithelium and/or the wall of the gall bladder (Fig. 5.34). In the acute stage the lesion can be associated with erosion and ulceration. In the chronic stage there is a mixed inflammatory infiltrate consisting of neutrophils, lymphocytes and plasma cells, and (possibly) fibrosis.

Lymphoplasmacellular and **follicular cholecystitis** is characterized by the presence of a lymphoplasmacytic infiltrate and/or the presence of lymphoid follicles in the mucosa of the gall bladder (Fig. 5.35).

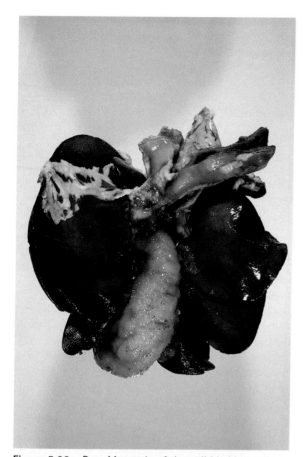

Figure 5.32 Dog. Mucocele of the gall bladder.

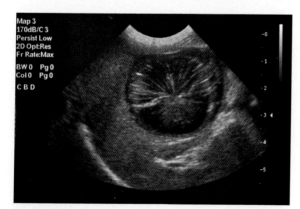

Figure 5.33 Ultrasonographic changes in a dog with gall bladder mucocele. The gall bladder is distended and contains thick mucinous material with a typical radiated structure mimicking a cross-section of an orange or kiwi fruit. (Reproduced with permission of Prof. P. Barthez, Department of Diagnostic Imaging, Faculty of Veterinary Medicine, University Utrecht).

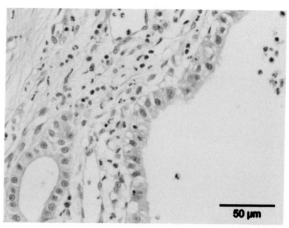

Figure 5.34 Dog. Neutrophilic cholangitis. HE.

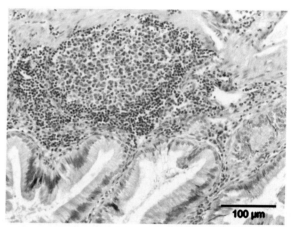

Figure 5.35 Dog. Lymphoplasmacellular and follicular cholecystitis. HE.

Infarction of the gall bladder

The gall bladder only has an arterial blood supply provided by the cystic artery, a branch of the hepatic artery. Occlusion of this branch by thrombosis may cause complete or partial infarction of the gall bladder as described in dogs.[29] The lesion is histologically characterized by full thickness necrosis of the wall of the gall bladder without evidence of concurrent cholecystitis (Fig. 5.36), and frequently, thrombosis of arteries.

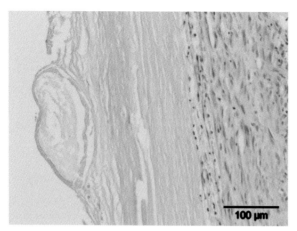

Figure 5.36 Dog. Infarction of the gall bladder. Full thickness necrosis of the wall of the gall bladder without inflammation; slight fibroblastic proliferation of the adnexal stroma. HE.

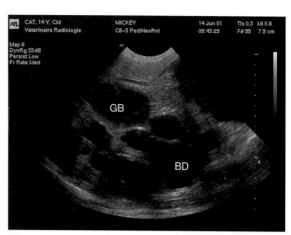

Figure 5.37 Ultrasonographic image of a cat with irregularly distended intra- and extrahepatic bile ducts due to lymphocytic cholangitis. Similar changes occur due to extrahepatic cholestasis and liver fluke infestation. GB – gall bladder; BD – bile duct. (Reproduced with permission of Dr George Voorhout, Department of Diagnostic Imaging, Faculty of Veterinary Medicine, University Utrecht).

ROLE OF HISTOPATHOLOGICAL EVALUATION, ULTRASONOGRAPHY AND EXAMINATION OF BILE IN THE DIAGNOSIS OF BILIARY DISORDERS

The diagnosis of biliary disorders depends often on a combination of different methods, unlike the parenchymal and neoplastic diseases, which are diagnosed exclusively by histopathological evaluation of the affected tissue. Intrahepatic cholestasis which is associated with many liver diseases is a pure histopathological finding. Cystic liver diseases are usually detected with ultrasonography, but the differentiation between different cystic lesions depends on histopathology. Extrahepatic bile duct obstruction leads to dilatation of the extrahepatic and intrahepatic bile ducts (dilatation of the gallbladder is not an essential feature), and is detected with ultrasonography. In dogs these ultrasonographic findings are diagnostic for extrahepatic cholestasis; the only disease with comparable ultrasound findings is Caroli's disease. However, extrahepatic cholestasis involves the large intrahepatic and extrahepatic ducts including the entire common bile duct, whereas Caroli's disease does not affect the common bile duct. These two possibilities can with certainty be differentiated with histopathological evaluation of the liver. In cats, neutrophilic cholangitis, lymphocytic cholangitis, cholangitis due to liver fluke infestation, and extra-

hepatic bile duct obstruction may have comparable ultrasonographic changes (Fig. 5.37). In all four diseases, ultrasonography may show dilatation of the entire biliary tree up to Vater's papilla. In cats it is therefore essential to sample liver tissue biopsies for histopathological differentiation of these four diseases. In cats with such lesions it is important to sample bile with puncture of the gallbladder with a thin needle for cytological evaluation and bacterial culture. The presence of neutrophils and the identification of bacteria in bile are essential in the diagnosis of neutrophilic cholangitis. Testing of sensitivity for antibiotics is essential for the appropriate treatment. This form of cholangitis in cats is usually acute without dilatation of the bile ducts and hence without the ultrasonographic changes seen in more chronic cases. Neutrophilic cholangitis does not always produce the typical histopathological changes and may not always be uniformly distributed throughout the liver; consequently the diagnosis may be missed when examination is limited to ultasonography and evaluation of a liver biopsy. Evaluation of the bile is required to make this diagnosis in cats that present with signs of nausea and vomiting and that may show

Table 5.2   The roles of histopathology, ultrasonography and bile sampling (cytological evaluation and culture) in the diagnosis of biliary diseases of dogs and cats

Disorder	Ultrasonography (A)	Histopathology of the liver (B)	Bile cytology (C)	Bile culture (D)	Minimal diagnostic requirement
Cystic diseases	+ or +/–	+	–	–	A and B
Extrahepatic cholestasis dog	+	+ or +/–	–	–	A
Extrahepatic cholestasis cat	+	+ or +/–	–	–	A,B,C, and D
Neutrophilic cholangitis	+/– or –	+/–	+	+	A,C, and D
Lymphocytic cholangitis	+	+	+/–	–	A,B,C, and D
Liver fluke infection	+	+	–	–	A, B,C and D
Destructive cholangitis	–	+	–	–	B
Gallbladder mucocele	+	–[a]	–	–	A

– = no changes demonstrated with this method
+/– = changes may be found, but may also be absent
+ = changes are always demonstrated
[a] Histopathology of the gallbladder required for final diagnosis

icterus and increased plasma bile acid and ALT or AP levels.[30–32]

DIAGNOSTIC TESTS REQUIRED FOR BILIARY DISEASES

The required diagnostic combinations for the biliary disorders of dogs and cats are summarized in Table 5.2.

SUMMARY

The biliary disorders can be grouped into four major categories:

1. Biliary cystic disease and biliary atresia
2. Cholestasis and cholatestasis
3. Cholangitis
4. Diseases of the gall bladder.

The biliary cystic diseases comprise solitary, usually acquired cysts and congenital cystic diseases. The latter are considered to be ductal plate anomalies and the various forms observed in dogs and cats correspond with those seen in humans and can be subdivided into three different subtypes, i.e. juvenile polycystic disease/congenital hepatic fibrosis, adult polycystic disease including Von Meyenburg complexes, and congenital dilatation of the large and segmental bile ducts. Extrahepatic biliary atresia is extremely rare and has been described only once in a dog. Cholestasis (bilirubinostasis) is morphologically characterized by the presence of bile in the hepatic parenchyma. Intrahepatic cholestasis is associated with a wide spectrum of liver diseases and microscopic lesions apart from the cholestasis are related to the primary hepatic disease. In extrahepatic cholestasis the lesions are related to the leakage of bile from the bile ducts into the connective tissue of the portal tracts, which causes an acute or chronic inflammation in the stromal tissue of these portal tracts; cholestasis is evident in acute cases but may be absent in chronic cases. Cholatestasis is characterized by swollen pale hepatocytes, preferentially in the periportal region, with centrally located, often coppercontaining granules. Cholangitis includes:

1. Neutrophilic cholangitis, usually resulting from a bacterial ascending infection
2. Lymphocytic cholangitis as observed in cats
3. Destructive cholangitis
4. Chronic cholangitis associated with liver fluke infestation.

Diseases of the gall bladder are cystic mucinous hyperplasia, neutrophilic and lymphoplasmacytic cholecystitis, and infarction of the gall bladder.

References

1. McSween RNM, Desmet VJ, Roskams T, et al. Developmental anatomy and normal structure. In: McSween RNM, Burt AD, Portmann BC, et al, eds. Pathology of the liver. 4th edn. London: Churchill Livingstone; 2002:3–66.

2. Cullen JM, MacLachlan NJ. Liver, biliary system and pancreas. In: McGavin MD, Carlton WW, Zachary JF, eds. Thomson's special veterinary pathology. St Louis; 2001:81–123.

3. Yamamoto K, Itoshima T, Tsuji T, et al. Three-dimensional fine structure of the biliary tract: scanning electron microscopy of biliary casts. J Electron Microsc Tech 1990; 14(3):208–217.

4. Portmann BC, Nakanuma Y. Diseases of the bile ducts. In: McSween RNM, Burt AD, Portmann BC, et al, eds. Pathology of the liver. 4th edn. London: Churchill Livingstone; 2002:435–506.

5. Rubarth S. Leber und Gallenwege. In: Dobberstein J, Pallaske G, Stünzi H, eds. Joest- Handbuch der Speziellen Pathologischen Anatomie der Haustiere. 3rd edn. Berlin: Paul Parey Verlag; 1967:1–177.

6. Desmet VJ. Congenital diseases of intrahepatic bile ducts: variation on a theme 'ductal plate malformation'. Hepatology 1992; 16:1069–1083.

7. Desmet VJ. Ludwig symposium on biliary disorders - part 1. Pathogenesis of ductal plate abnormalities. Mayo Clin Proc 1998; 73:80–89.

8. van Eijken P, Sciot R, Van der Steen K, et al. The development of the intrahepatic bile ducts in man: a keratin immunohistochemical study. Hepatology 1988; 8:1586–1595.

9. Desmet VJ. Embryology of the liver and intrahepatic biliary tract, and an overview of malformations of the bile ducts. In: Macintire N, Benhamou J-P, Bircher J, et al, eds. Oxford textbook of clinical hepatology. Oxford: Oxford University Press; 1991:495–519.

10. Libbrecht L, Cassiman D, Desmet V, et al. The correlation between portal myofibroblasts and development of intrahepatic bile ducts and arterial branches in human liver. Liver 2002; 22(3):252–257.

11. Ishak KG, Sharp HL. Developmental abnormalities and liver disease in childhood. In: McSween RNM, Burt AD, Portmann BC, et al, eds. Pathology of the liver. 4th edn. London: Churchill Livingstone; 2002:107–154.

12. Crawford JM. The Liver. In: Cotran RS, Kumar V, Collins T, eds. Robbins pathologic basis of disease. 6th edn. Philadelphia: W.B. Saunders; 1999:846–890.

13. van den Ingh TS, Rothuizen J. Congenital cystic disease of the liver in seven dogs. J Comp Pathol 1985; 95(3):405–414.

14. Görlinger S, Rothuizen J, Bunch SE, et al. Congenital dilatation of the bile ducts (Caroli's disease) in young dogs. J Vet Intern Med 2003; 17:28–32.

15. Bosje JT, van den Ingh TS, van der Linde-Sipman JS. Polycystic kidney and liver disease in cats. Vet Q 1998; 20(4):136–139.

16. Schulze C, Rothuizen J, van Sluijs FJ, et al. Extrahepatic biliary atresia in a border collie. J Small Anim Pract 2000; 41(1):27–30.

17. Raweily EA, Gibson AAM, Burt AD. Abnormalities of intrahepatic bile ducts in extrahepatic biliary atresia. Histopathology 1990; 17:521–527.

18. Low Y, Vijanyan V, Tan CE. The prognostic significance of ductal plate malformation and other histologic parameters in biliary atresia: an immunohistochemical study. J Pediatr 2001; 139:320–322.

19. van den Ingh TS, Rothuizen J, van den Brom WE. Extrahepatic cholestasis in the dog and the differentiation of extrahepatic and intrahepatic cholestasis. Vet Q 1986; 8(2): 150–157.

20. Day DG. Feline cholangiohepatitis complex. Vet Clin North Am Small Anim Pract 1995; 25(2):375–385.

21. Gagne JM, Weiss DJ, Armstrong PJ. Histopathologic evaluation of feline inflammatory liver disease. Vet Pathol 1996; 33:521–526.

22. Weiss DJ, Armstrong PJ, Gagne J. Inflammatory liver disease. Semin Vet Med Surg (Small Anim) 1997; 12(1):22–27.

23. Lucke VM, Davies JD. Progressive lymphocytic cholangitis in the cat. J Small Anim Pract 1984; 25:249–260.

24. van den Ingh TS, Rothuizen J, van Zinnicq Bergman HM. Destructive cholangiolitis in seven dogs. Vet Q 1988; 10(4):240–245.

25. Wetzel R. Parasitäre Erkrankungen der Leber und der Gallenwege. In: Dobberstein J, Pallaske G, Stünzi H, editors. Joest- Handbuch der Speziellen Pathologischen Anatomie der Haustiere. 3rd edn. Berlin: Paul Parey Verlag; 1967:209–299.

26. Bowman DD, Hendrix CM, Lindsay DS, et al. Feline clinical parasitology. 1st edn. Ames: Iowa State University Press; 2002.

27. Pike FS, Berg J, King NW, et al. Gallbladder mucocele in dogs: 30 cases (2000–2002). J Am Vet Med Assoc 2004; 224(10):1615–1622.

28. Besso JG, Wrigley RH, Gliatto JM, et al. Ultrasonographic appearance and clinical findings in

14 dogs with gallbladder mucocele. Vet Radiol Ultrasound 2000; 41(3):261–271.

29. Holt DE, Mehler S, Mayhew PD, et al. Canine gallbladder infarction: 12 cases (1993–2003). Vet Pathol 2004; 41:416–418.

30. Gagne JM, Armstrong PJ, Weiss DJ, et al. Clinical features of inflammatory liver disease in cats: 41 cases (1983–1993). J Am Vet Med Assoc 1999; 214(4):513–516.

31. Newell SM, Selcer BA, Girard E, et al. Correlations between ultrasonographic findings and specific hepatic diseases in cats: 72 cases (1985–1997). J Am Vet Med Assoc 1998; 213(1):94–98.

32. Center SA, Baldwin BH, Erb H, et al. Bile acid concentrations in the diagnosis of hepatobiliary disease in the cat. J Am Vet Med Assoc 1986; 189(8):891–896.

Chapter **6**

Morphological classification of parenchymal disorders of the canine and feline liver

1. Normal histology, reversible hepatocytic injury and hepatic amyloidosis

John M. Cullen, Ted S. G. A. M. van den Ingh, Tom Van Winkle, Jenny A. Charles, Valeer J. Desmet

INTRODUCTION

The normal histology of the smallest liver unit and the normal features of its constituent components are described in order to recognize the various parenchymal disorders and to understand the terminology used. The parenchymal disorders can be grouped into seven categories:

1. Reversible hepatocellular injury: cell swelling, steroid-induced hepatopathy and steatosis (syn. lipidosis) (this chapter)
2. Hepatic amyloidosis (this chapter)
3. Hepatocellular death: apoptosis and necrosis (Ch. 7)
4. Acute and chronic hepatitis and cirrhosis (Ch. 7)
5. Hepatic abscesses and granulomas (Ch. 8)
6. Hepatic metabolic storage diseases (Ch. 8)
7. Miscellaneous conditions (Ch. 8).

Histological examination of liver biopsies can substantially aid in the diagnosis of all categories of parenchymal disease. Changes in the hepatocytes are the hallmarks of most of these disorders. However, these hepatocytic changes, as well as other primary or secondary lesions such as inflammation, fibrosis, and bile duct proliferation, are not restricted to parenchymal disorders and may be

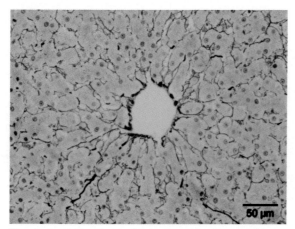

Figure 6.1 Cat. Terminal hepatic vein with radiating reticulin network. Gordon and Sweet stain for reticulin.

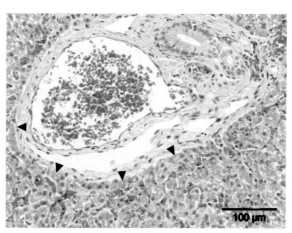

Figure 6.2 Dog. Normal portal area with limiting plate (arrowheads). HE.

present in primary biliary and circulatory disorders. Differentiation of these disorders is usually possible through careful histological examination and evaluation of the combination of the parenchymal, vascular and portal lesions present in the affected liver.

NORMAL HISTOLOGY OF THE LIVER PARENCHYMA

The parenchyma consists of hepatic cords/plates and sinusoids. The hepatic cords/plates are usually one cell thick and have a regular arrangement around the central (terminal) hepatic vein causing a radiating pattern of the sinusoidal network and the accompanying reticulin framework (Fig. 6.1); outside the perivenular zone the cords/plates are less regularly arranged, with loss of the radiating pattern. The hepatocytes situated at the periphery of the classical lobule form the so-called limiting plate, which is well demarcated from the adjacent stromal tissue of the portal tract (Fig. 6.2). Individual hepatocytes are polygonal and have a pale to eosinophilic cytoplasm, depending on the quantity of cytoplasmic glycogen, and clearly outlined cell margins. The nucleus is centrally placed and one or more nucleoli may be recognized; binucleated cells may occasionally be found. Mitoses, even in biopsy material, are rarely seen. The sinusoids form an apparently discontinuous system of narrow channels between the liver cell cords/plates and are

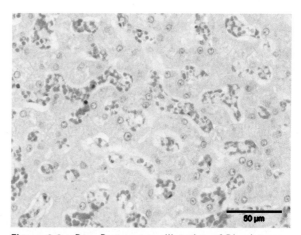

Figure 6.3 Dog. Postmortem dilatation of Disse's space and separation of sinusoidal lining cells and Kupffer cells from the hepatic cords. HE.

covered by fenestrated endothelium. In the normal biopsy the lining cells are inconspicuous except for their flattened elongated nuclei. Kupffer cells (hepatic macrophages) are more plump cells, often containing some ceroid pigment, and extend to the lumen of the sinusoids. The perisinusoidal space of Disse is not recognized in biopsy material, but in postmortem material becomes dilated and sinusoidal lining cells and Kupffer cells appear to separate from the adjacent hepatocytes (Fig. 6.3). The hepatic stellate cells (also known as: Ito cells, fat storing cells, lipocytes) are located in the space of

Disse, randomly distributed in the lobules, and can be identified by the presence of small or large fat droplets (see Fig. 8.22).[1] Hepatic stellate cells are important for the liver function as:

- They produce the extracellular matrix in the normal and diseased liver; in response to stimulation by cytokines they become activated with a myofibroblastic appearance and will cause increased deposition of extracellular matrix and thus contribute to fibrosis
- They act in a pericyte like manner around the sinusoids, regulating the sinusoidal blood flow
- They are a major site of vitamin A storage
- They may play a role in hepatic regeneration as they express hepatocytic growth factor (HGF).[2]

The hepatic parenchyma has been described as being arranged in either lobules or acini and both concepts and related terminologies are used in literature (Fig. 6.4). The classic hepatic lobule is a hexagonal structure arranged around the central vein and bordered at its periphery by multiple portal areas. In the lobular concept the centrilobular area is the parenchymal zone closest to the central vein, the periportal area is the zone adjacent to the portal area and the midzonal area is the parenchyma between these two. The liver can also be viewed as containing acinar units with the terminal hepatic arterioles and portal veins radiating from the portal area forming the central axis of the acinus with the terminal hepatic veins (central veins) at the periphery. In the acinar concept the parenchyma adjacent to the terminal hepatic arteriole and portal vein is referred to as periportal or acinar zone 1. The parenchyma adjacent to the terminal hepatic vein is referred to as perivenous or acinar zone 3, whereas the area in between is called acinar zone 2.[1]

CLASSIFICATION OF PARENCHYMAL DISORDERS

Reversible hepatocytic injury

Hepatocellular swelling, steroid-induced hepatopathy and steatosis (syn. lipidosis) are patterns of reversible cell injury of the liver. Generally, they are characterized by focal or diffuse swelling, a focal, zonal or diffuse pale or yellow-tan discoloration,

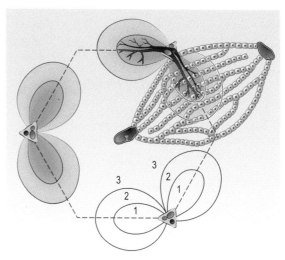

Figure 6.4   *Schematic presentation of the classic hexagonal lobule and the simple acinus of Rappaport.*

and a decreased consistency with increased fragility of the liver.

Hepatocellular swelling

Hepatocellular swelling (also known as: cloudy swelling, hydropic degeneration) is the first manifestation of almost all forms of injury to cells and appears whenever cells are incapable of maintaining ionic and fluid homeostasis, and consequently accumulate water. Mild to moderate hepatocellular swelling is a difficult morphological change to appreciate with the light microscope. In more advanced cases the hepatocytes will show a more severe hydropic change with marked swelling and pale staining cytoplasm arranged in thin strands, or vacuolar change of the cytoplasm. Ultrastructural changes include plasma membrane alterations (blebbing, blunting and distortion of microvilli, formation of myelin figures and loosening of intercellular attachments), mitochondrial changes (swelling, rarefaction and appearance of amorphous densities), dilation of the endoplasmic reticulum with detachment and disaggregation of polysomes, and nuclear alterations.[3]

Feathery degeneration is a form of hydropic degeneration of hepatocytes associated with cholestasis and is most likely caused by the intracellular accumulation of bilirubin and bile acids.

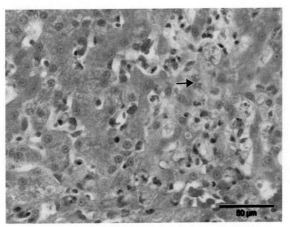

Figure 6.5   Dog. Feathery degeneration and a bile lake (arrow). HE.

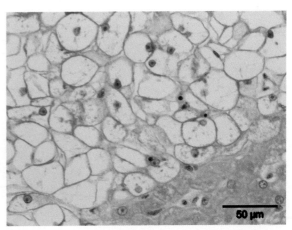

Figure 6.6   Dog. Steroid-induced hepatopathy. HE.

The lesion is characterized by enlarged hepatocytes with pale staining cytoplasm arranged in thin strands in combination with the intracytoplasmic presence of bilirubin (Fig. 6.5) and may precede the formation of bile-infarcts.[4,5] Bilirubin is often difficult to demonstrate with light microscopy and is more readily seen with electron microscopy. The lesion is particularly seen in severe extrahepatic cholestasis and in destructive cholangitis.

Steroid-induced hepatopathy

Steroid-induced hepatopathy is a specific disorder in dogs characterized by excessive hepatocellular glycogen accumulation.[6,7] The characteristic features are swollen hepatocytes with clear cytoplasm and strands of eosinophilic cytoplasm without displacement of the nucleus from the center (Fig. 6.6). The distribution and the extent of the lesion varies markedly and can be diffuse, zonal or involve small groups or even individual cells. Periodic acid Schiff (PAS) staining with or without diastase may help to identify the glycogen accumulation; frozen sections are the most suitable method for the demonstration of glycogen. Other hepatic changes seen in association with steroid-induced hepatopathy are marginated neutrophils in small blood vessels and occasional foci of extramedullary myelopoiesis. Fragmentation of needle biopsies is common in livers with marked steroid-induced hepatopathy.

Although usually induced by either exogenous (iatrogenic hypercorticism) or endogenous glucocorticoids (pituitary-dependent hyperadrenocorticism and hyperadrenocorticism due to adrenocortical tumors), there are anecdotal reports that other steroid hormones (progestins and aldosterone) and drugs (e.g. D-penicillamine) may induce these changes. Sometimes dogs with well-documented spontaneous hyperadrenocorticism do not have this change.

Hepatocellular steatosis (lipidosis, fatty change)

These terms (lipidosis, steatosis, fatty change or fatty liver) are used interchangeably by some, but others have strong opinions about the use of these terms. Common textbooks in human pathology[3,8,9] and toxicological pathology[10] use steatosis (syn. lipidosis) and fatty change interchangeably, while veterinary textbooks,[11–14] and other toxicological pathology texts[15] tend to use fatty change and lipidosis interchangeably. Clinicians should recognize that pathologists will continue to use steatosis, lipidosis and fatty change (fatty liver) to mean the same change inhepatocytes.

Hepatocellular steatosis is the accumulation of lipid-containing vacuoles within the cytoplasm of hepatocytes. In routine formalin-fixed, paraffin-embedded material the fat is seen as clear, empty vacuoles since the lipid is lost during processing.

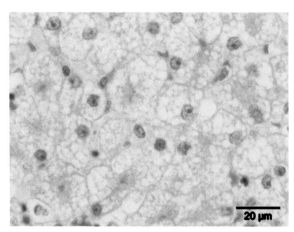

Figure 6.7   Dog. Microvesicular steatosis (syn. lipidosis). Juvenile hypoglycaemia. HE.

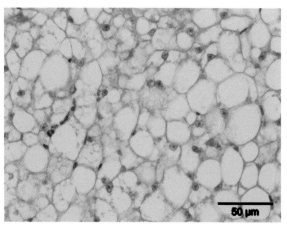

Figure 6.8   Cat. Macro- and microvesicular steatosis (syn. lipidosis). Feline hepatic lipidosis. HE.

Lipid can be demonstrated in frozen sections using Oil Red O or Sudan black, or in tissue that has been postfixed in osmium tetroxide. Two major patterns of steatosis (syn. lipidosis) are recognized on light microscopy: microvesicular and macrovesicular steatosis (syn. lipidosis). In microvesicular steatosis (syn. lipidosis), the hepatocytic cytoplasm is filled with vacuoles, which are uniform in size and smaller than the centrally located nucleus (Fig. 6.7). Microvesicular steatosis (syn. lipidosis) is typically seen in dogs with diabetes mellitus,[6] in which the lipid accumulation begins in the centrilobular areas, and in juvenile hypoglycemia of small breed dogs[16] in which the accumulation may be diffuse or centrilobular. In macrovesicular steatosis (syn. lipidosis) the cytoplasmic vacuoles are the size of the nucleus or larger and the vacuoles may displace the nucleus to the periphery of the cell. In cats affected with the syndrome of feline hepatic lipidosis, a severe diffuse form of hepatic steatosis (syn. lipidosis), a mixed form, is seen where the hepatocytes show multiple vacuoles of different size (Figs 6.8, 6.9). Hepatocellular steatosis (syn. lipidosis) should not be confused with accumulation of lipid in hepatic stellate cells (see Miscellaneous Conditions).

Hepatocellular steatosis (syn. lipidosis) is a nonspecific reversible form of cellular injury and different mechanisms account for triglyceride (triacylglycerol) accumulation in the liver. Free fatty acids from adipose tissue or ingested food are nor-

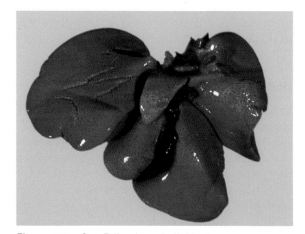

Figure 6.9   Cat. Feline hepatic lipidosis.

mally transported into hepatocytes. In the liver, they are esterified to triacylglycerol, converted into cholesterol or phospholipids, or oxidized to ketone bodies. Release of triacylglycerols from the hepatocytes requires association with apoproteins to form lipoproteins, which are released into the circulation. Steatosis (syn. lipidosis) may result from defects in any of the events in this sequence and includes:

- Excessive transport of fatty acids into the liver from dietary intake of fat or carbohydrates or from mobilization of triglycerids from the adipose tissue (starvation, diabetes mellitus)

- Abnormal hepatocyte function with decreased energy for oxidation of fatty acids (hypoxia) or toxic damage to mitochondria (tetracycline)
- Increased esterification of fatty acids to triglycerids in response to increased amounts of glucose and insulin (hyperadrenocorticism)
- Decreased apoprotein synthesis (dietary deficiency, hepatotoxins and toxic drugs)
- Impaired secretion of lipoproteins from the liver caused by secretory defects (hepatotoxins and toxic drugs).[12]

As various causes may have a different type and distribution of the lesion and severe steatosis (syn. lipidosis) may affect the function of the liver, it is necessary to communicate to the clinician not only the type of vacuolation but also the severity and the distribution (focal, periportal, centrilobular, diffuse) of the steatosis (syn. lipidosis), as well as other possible hepatic lesions which may give a clue to the underlying disease mechanism.

Hepatic amyloidosis

Amyloid in the liver of dogs and cats is usually secondary or reactive amyloid [serum amyloid-associated (SAA) protein] and deposition occurs as a consequence of long-standing inflammation or tissue destruction and the production by the liver of its precursor, the acute phase protein serum amyloid A. Histologically, it appears as deposition of hyaline eosinophilic material in the space of Disse frequently associated with atrophy of the adjacent hepatocytes (Fig. 6.10) and, particularly in needle biopsies, dilation of sinusoids. The amyloid deposition may have a diffuse, zonal, or multifocal parenchymal distribution and may be accompanied by deposition of amyloid in the wall of vessels and in the portal and perivenular connective tissue. Special stains (Congo red or Stokes) may be needed to identify or confirm the presence of amyloid (Fig. 6.11). With extensive hepatic accumulation of amyloid the liver becomes markedly enlarged and fragile, and intrahepatic haemorrhage as well as spontaneous or biopsy-induced liver rupture with hemorrhage and hemoabdomen may occur (Fig. 6.12).[17,18]

Hepatic amyloidosis is commonly associated with inflammatory conditions in other organ

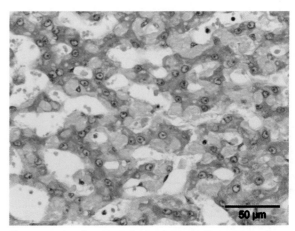

Figure 6.10 Cat. Hepatic amyloidosis. Deposition of hyaline eosinophilic material in the space of Disse with atrophy of the hepatocytes. HE.

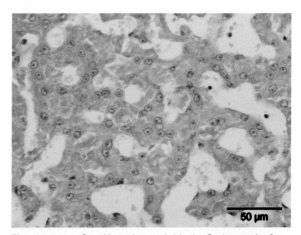

Figure 6.11 Cat. Hepatic amyloidosis. Stokes stain for amyloid.

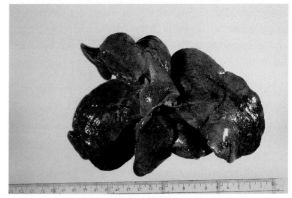

Figure 6.12 Cat. Hepatic amyloidosis with subcapsular haemorrhage due to fragility of the liver.

systems; however, in breeds with a familial predisposition to amyloidosis (Chinese Shar-pei dogs[19] and Abyssinian,[20,21] Siamese and other Oriental cats[22,23]) inflammation in other organs may be slight or negligible.

SUMMARY

The normal anatomy of the classical liver lobule and acinus of Rappaport and the constituent elements of the hepatic parenchyma, i.e. the hepatocytes, sinusoids, Kupffer cells and hepatic stellate cells are described. The parenchymal disorders of the liver in dogs and cats mentioned in this chapter are hepatic amyloidosis and the various forms of reversible hepatocellular injury, i.e. hepatocellular swelling, feathery degeneration, steroid-induced hepatopathy and steatosis (syn. lipidosis).

References

1. McSween RNM, Desmet VJ, Roskams T, et al. Developmental anatomy and normal structure. In: McSween RNM, Burt AD, Portmann BC, et al, eds. Pathology of the liver. 4th edn. London: Churchill Livingstone; 2002:3–66.
2. Bedossa P, Paradis V. Liver extracellular matrix in health and disease. J Pathol 2003; 200:504–515.
3. Cotran RS, Kumar V, Collins T. Robbins: pathologic basis of disease. Philadelphia: WB Saunders; 2000.
4. Poulsen H, Christoffersen P. Atlas of liver biopsies. 1st edn. Copenhagen: Munksgaard; 1979.
5. Portmann BC, Nakanuma Y. Diseases of the bile ducts. In: McSween RNM, Burt AD, Portmann BC, et al, eds. Pathology of the liver. 4th edn. London: Churchill Livingstone; 2002:435–506.
6. Lettow E, Loppnow H. Funktionelle und morphologische Untersuchungen der Leber bei Hunden mit manifestem und latentem Diabetes mellitus. In: Gaines European Veterinary Symposium; 1972 June 3; Amsterdam: Gaines; 1972:25–28.
7. Badylak SF, Van Vleet JF. Tissue gamma-glutamyl transpeptidase activity and hepatic ultrastructural alterations in dogs with experimentally induced glucocorticoid hepatopathy. Am J Vet Res 1982; 43(4):649–655.
8. Burt AD, Portmann BC, McSween RNM. Liver pathology associated with diseases of other organs or systems. In: McSween RNM, Burt AD, Portmann BC, et al, eds. Pathology of the liver. 4th edn. Edinburgh: Churchill Livingstone; 2002.
9. Rubin E, Farber JL. Pathology. 3rd edn. Philadelphia: Lippincott Raven; 1999.
10. Greaves P. Histopathology of preclinical toxicity studies. 2nd edn. Amsterdam: Elsevier; 2000.
11. Kelly WR. The liver and biliary system. In: Jubb KVF, Kennedy PC, Palmer N, eds. Pathology of domestic animals. 4th edn. San Diego: Academic Press; 1992:319–406.
12. Cullen JM, MacLachlan NJ. Liver, biliary system and pancreas. In: McGavin MD, Carlton WW, Zachary JF, eds. Thomson's special veterinary pathology. St Louis; 2001:81–123.
13. Percy DH, Barthold SW. Pathology of laboratory rodents and rabbits. Ames: Iowa State University Press; 1993.
14. Jones TC, Hunt RD, King NW. Veterinary Pathology. 6th edn. Baltimore: Williams and Wilkins; 1997.
15. Haschek WM, Rousseaux CG. Handbook of toxicologic pathology. San Diego: Academic Press; 1991.
16. Van der Linde-Sipman JS, Van den Ingh TSGAM, Van Toor AJ. Fatty liver syndrome in puppies. J Am Anim Hosp Assoc 1990; 26:9–12.
17. Beatty JA, Barrs VR, Martin PA, et al. Spontaneous hepatic rupture in six cats with systemic amyloidosis. J Small Anim Pract 2002; 43(8):355–363.
18. Godfrey DR, Day MJ. Generalised amyloidosis in two Siamese cats: spontaneous liver haemorrhage and chronic renal failure. J Small Anim Pract 1998; 39(9):442–447.
19. DiBartola SP, Tarr MJ, Webb DM, et al. Familial renal amyloidosis in Chinese Shar Pei dogs. J Am Vet Med Assoc 1990; 197(4):483–487.
20. DiBartola SP, Hill RL, Fechheimer NS, et al. Pedigree analysis of Abyssinian cats with familial amyloidosis. Am J Vet Res 1986; 47(12):2666–2668.
21. Boyce JT, DiBartola SP, Chew DJ, et al. Familial renal amyloidosis in Abyssinian cats. Vet Pathol 1984; 21(1):33–38.
22. van der Linde-Sipman JS, Niewold TA, Tooten PC, de Neijs-Backer M, Gruys E. Generalized AA-amyloidosis in Siamese and Oriental cats. Vet Immunol Immunopathol 1997;56(1-2):1-10.
23. Niewold TA, van der Linde-Sipman JS, Murphy C, Tooten PC, Gruys E. Familial amyloidosis in cats: Siamese and Abyssinian AA proteins differ in primary sequence and pattern of deposition. Amyloid 1999;6(3):205-9.

Chapter **7**

Morphological classification of parenchymal disorders of the canine and feline liver

2. Hepatocellular death, hepatitis and cirrhosis

Ted S. G. A. M. van den Ingh, Tom Van Winkle,
John M. Cullen, Jenny A. Charles, Valeer J. Desmet

HEPATOCELLULAR DEATH: APOPTOSIS AND NECROSIS

Hepatocytes may be killed by various insults including hypoxia, toxins, microorganisms, immunological events and severe metabolic disturbances. Classically, cell death has been considered to occur through apoptosis or necrosis; however, recent evidence suggests overlap between both processes as moderate exposure to some toxins causes apoptosis whereas greater exposure may result in necrosis[1,2] and that necrosis and apoptosis are morphological expressions of a shared biochemical network of both caspase-dependent mechanisms as well as non-caspase-dependent effectors.[2] **Apoptosis** is a caspase-dependent active process of programmed cell death which results in shrinkage of the cell without loss of integrity of the cell and nuclear membrane, and subsequent fragmentation and phagocytosis of these fragments by neighboring Kupffer cells and hepatocytes (Fig. 7.1).[3] **Necrosis** involves cytoplasmic swelling and loss of integrity of the cell membrane and may result in coagulative necrosis or liquefactive (lytic) necrosis. **Coagulative necrosis** is the result of sudden and catastrophic denaturation of the cytosolic protein and appears as swollen hepatocytes with acidophilic cytoplasm, preservation of the basic outline of the coagulated cell, and

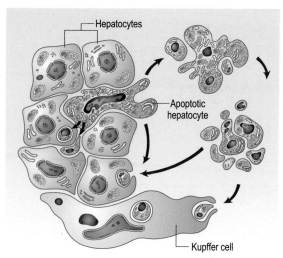

Figure 7.1 Schematic presentation of hepatocellular apoptosis (shrinkage necrosis) with subsequent fragmentation and phagocytosis of the fragments by adjacent hepatocytes and Kupffer cells.

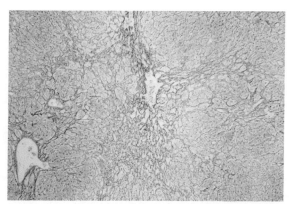

Figure 7.3 Liquefactive necrosis as evidenced by loss of hepatocytes and collapse of the residual reticulin network. Gordon and Sweet stain for reticulin.

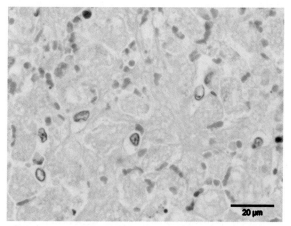

Figure 7.2 Coagulative necrosis of the hepatocytes with slight proliferation of Kupffer cells. HE.

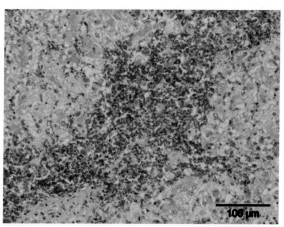

Figure 7.4 Liquefactive necrosis as evidenced by loss of hepatocytes and replacement by erythrocytes. HE.

karyopyknosis, karyorrhexis or karyolysis (Fig. 7.2). The acute phase of coagulative necrosis is followed by proliferation of Kupffer cells and infiltration of mononuclear and polymorphonuclear phagocytes and subsequent resorbtion and lysis of the necrotic cells. **Liquefactive** or **lytic necrosis** is the result of osmotic swelling and disintegration of hepatocytes and appears as loss of hepatocytes with subsequent collapse of the residual reticulin network (Fig. 7.3) and/or replacement by erythrocytes (Fig. 7.4) and eventually the presence of ceroid-laden macrophages (Fig. 7.5). The outcome of a given hepatic insult depends on the nature, extent and duration of the insult, and of course survival of the host.

Morphological patterns of apoptosis and necrosis[4-6]

Apoptotic body (acidophil body)

Apoptotic hepatocytes are shrunken, intensely eosinophilic cells with condensed nuclei and they

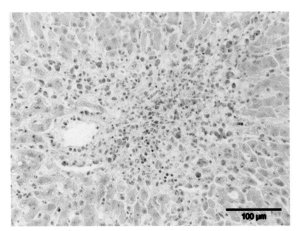

Figure 7.5   Liquefactive necrosis as evidenced by loss of hepatocytes and presence of ceroid-laden macrophages. HE.

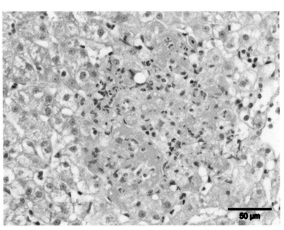

Figure 7.7   Focal necrosis with reactive Kupffer cell proliferation and infiltration of mononuclear and polymorphonuclear phagocytes. HE.

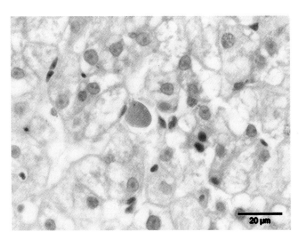

Figure 7.6   Apoptotic (acidophil) body.

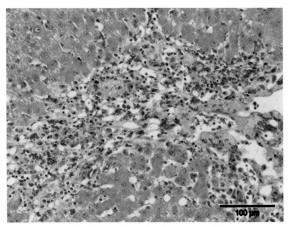

Figure 7.8   Confluent liquefactive necrosis in the acinar periphery with collapse and ceroid-laden macrophages. HE.

are surrounded by an empty halo (Fig. 7.6) After subsequent fragmentation, the remnants are phagocytosed by adjacent Kupffer cells and hepatocytes, and are visible as small cytoplasmic eosinophilic inclusions that are rapidly degraded.

Focal and multifocal necrosis

These terms refer to coagulative or liquefactive necrosis of small aggregates of hepatocytes, mostly attended and recognized by the secondary inflammatory reaction of Kupffer cell proliferation and infiltration of mononuclear and/or polymorphonuclear phagocytes (Fig. 7.7).

Confluent and bridging necrosis

Confluent necrosis may be coagulative or liquefactive necrosis and comprises larger areas of hepatocytes, in a random or zonal distribution (Fig. 7.8). Confluent necrosis linking vascular structures is called bridging necrosis. Bridging at the periphery of acini links terminal hepatic venules to each other and is called central-central bridging (Figs 7.9, 7.10, 7.11). Bridging linking terminal hepatic venules and portal tracts is called central-portal bridging, whereas bridging necrosis with a

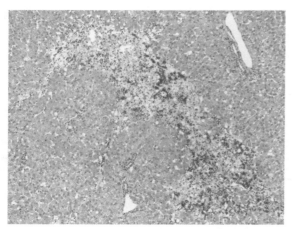

Figure 7.9   Central-central bridging liquefactive necrosis. HE.

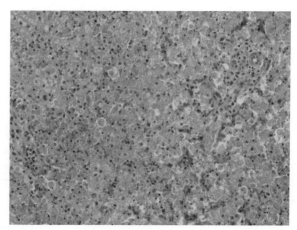

Figure 7.12   Diffuse panlobular to multilobular coagulative necrosis. Amanitum intoxication. HE.

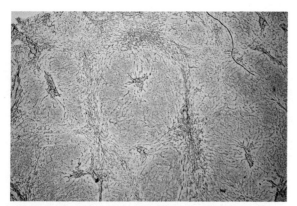

Figure 7.10   Central-central and slight central-portal liquefactive necrosis as evidenced by collapse of the reticulin network. Gordon and Sweet stain for reticulin.

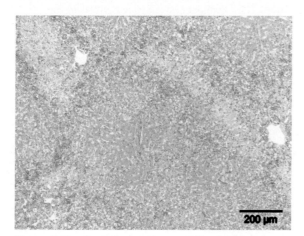

Figure 7.11   Central-central coagulative bridging necrosis. HE.

periportal distribution is called portal-portal bridging. When confluent necrosis is more extensive and involves complete acini or lobules, the process is described as panacinar or panlobular necrosis (Fig. 7.12).

Massive necrosis

This form of necrosis is the most severe form and generally applies when the liver shows extensive diffuse panlobular and multilobular coagulative and/or liqueactive necrosis (Fig. 7.13). The sequel of massive necrosis is often collapse of the reticulin and fibrous network so that portal areas and hepatic venules come more closely together due to the loss of intermediate tissue in the lobule. The connective tissue subsequently condenses (postnecrotic scarring).

Piecemeal necrosis

Piecemeal necrosis, recently called **interface hepatitis,**[4] can be defined as death of hepatocytes at the interface of parenchyma and (newly formed) connective tissue. The most likely process involved is apoptotis. The lesion is characterized by a variable degree of mononuclear inflammation and mostly fibrosis of the portal areas with infiltration and destruction of the limiting plate; sometimes apoptotic bodies can be observed in these areas (Fig. 7.14).

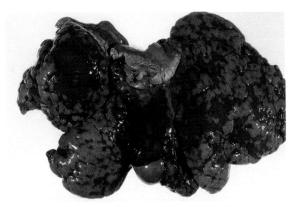

Figure 7.13   Dog. Massive hepatic necrosis (fulminant hepatitis) with collapsed dark-red areas.

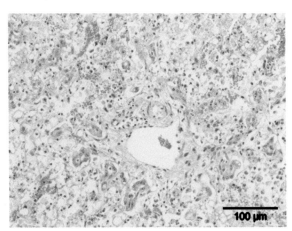

Figure 7.15   Extensive hepatocellular necrosis with proliferation of ductular structures in the periportal areas. HE.

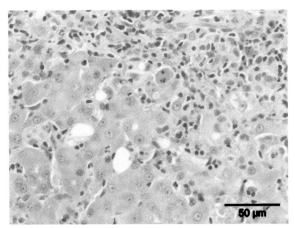

Figure 7.14   Interface hepatitis with infiltration and destruction of the limiting plate and some apoptotic bodies. HE.

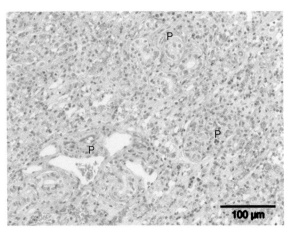

Figure 7.16   Postnecrotic scarring with approximation of portal areas (P) and periportal ductular proliferation. HE.

RESPONSE OF THE LIVER TO HEPATOCELLULAR INJURY

Following destruction of hepatic parenchyma, regeneration of parenchyma, fibrosis, and ductular proliferation may occur. When hepatocytic destruction is limited and the reticulin network remains intact, regeneration with almost complete restitution of the liver structure can occur through mitotic division of neighboring hepatocytes. Severe parenchymal destruction with extensive loss of hepatocytes is often followed by ductular proliferation. Many of these structures contain both liver cell and bile duct elements and may reflect regenerative proliferation of a hepatic stem cell popula-

tion analogous to oval cells in the rat, or transformation of regenerating hepatocytes into ductular structures. These structures are generally most prominent in the periportal areas, and their location corresponds to the former canals of Hering which are transformed into complex arborizing networks of proliferating cells (Fig. 7.15). With persistent parenchymal damage or extensive loss of hepatocytes fibrosis and postnecrotic scarring (Figs 7.16, 7.17) may occur with the formation of intrahepatic portovenous shunts; in these cases

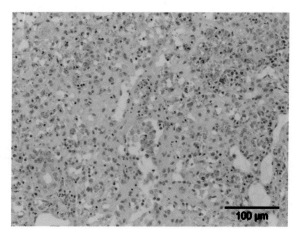

Figure 7.17 Postnecrotic scarring with fibrosis and a moderate inflammatory infiltrate of (ceroid-laden) macrophages, lymphocytes and plasma cells. HE.

prolonged regenerative effort will result in regenerative parenchymal nodules.

TOXIC LIVER INJURY

The liver is a common site of toxic injury as it receives blood from the portal system so that ingested toxins may cause direct hepatic injury at first passage or after metabolic transformation by the liver from non-toxic substances to toxic metabolites. Toxins are often plant and fungal products, drugs or chemicals, and may cause a predictable dose-dependent injury or an idiosyncratic non-dose dependent reaction in a minority of exposed animals. Mechanisms of hepatotoxicity include: alkylation of DNA (cyclophosphamide, pyrrolizidine alkaloids) or intercalation into DNA (actinomycin), binding to RNA polymerase (amanitin, a mushroom toxin), impaired RNA transcription (aflatoxin) or interference with ribosomal translation (ethionine). Toxins may also affect lysosomes by inhibiting lysosomal enzymes (e.g. mannosidosis induced by locoweed poisoning), or cause direct cell membrane damage through the generation of free radicals (vitamin E – selenium – fatty acid imbalance, CCL4, and bacterial toxins).

Toxic hepatic injury varies considerably with the type of reaction, dose and duration of exposure to the toxin. Manifestations of toxic hepatic injury, one or more of which may occur with any toxin, include: no morphological abnormalities (bio-chemical alterations only), hepatocellular swelling, steatosis and necrosis – usually in a specific pattern (centrilobular, periportal, midzonal or massive), cholestasis, inflammation and fibrosis. Although there may be anamnestic or histological clues suggesting toxic injury, it is very difficult to distinguish a cause of acute or chronic liver injury by morphological means alone.

HEPATITIS AND CIRRHOSIS

There is an intricate relationship between inflammation in the liver parenchyma and hepatocellular apoptosis and necrosis, the latter often being the initiating event of the inflammation. Nevertheless, considerable controversy exists about the preferred nomenclature in cases of acute hepatic necrosis in non-infectious, particularly toxic or ischemic insults, i.e. acute hepatic necrosis versus acute hepatitis. However, infectious causes of hepatocellular necrosis, traditionally referred to as hepatitis, may also show extensive hepatic necrosis with minimal, or even without, inflammation in the acute stage. No disagreement exists about the term chronic hepatitis, which is used irrespective of the cause, and which is characterized by the presence of fibrosis, inflammation and hepatocellular apoptosis and necrosis. The Working Group agreed that, irrespective of the nomenclature used, a morphological diagnosis should emphasize the type, pattern and extent of the necrosis and inflammation and the possible cause, as well as in more prolonged disease, the presence, pattern and extent of fibrosis and regeneration.

Acute hepatitis

General

Acute hepatitis is characterized morphologically by a combination of inflammation, hepatocellular apoptosis and necrosis, and in some instances, regeneration (Figs 7.18, 7.19). The proportion and detailed nature of these components vary widely according to the cause, the host response and the passage of time, and it is necessary to include in the diagnosis the type, pattern and extent of the necrosis and inflammation as well as the possible etiology. The lesions are usually suffi-

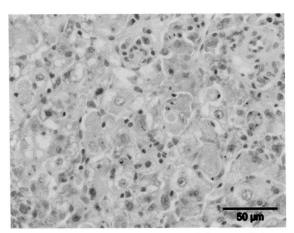

Figure 7.18   Dog. Acute hepatitis with hepatocellular necrosis and inflammation. HE.

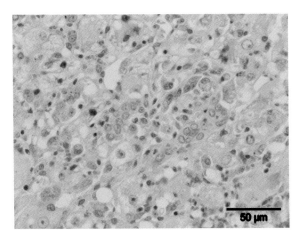

Figure 7.19   Dog. Acute hepatitis with inflammation and ductular proliferation. HE.

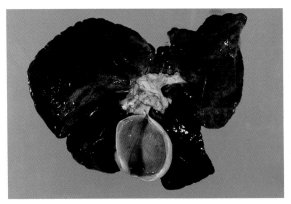

Figure 7.20   Canine contagious hepatitis due to adenovirus type 1 infection. Dark mottled appearance of the liver and characteristic edema of the wall of the gall bladder.

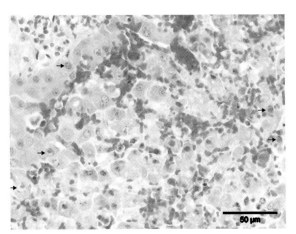

Figure 7.21   Canine contagious hepatitis due to adenovirus type 1 infection. Severe centrolobular necrosis and presence of intranuclear basophilic viral inclusions (arrows). HE.

ciently diffuse within the liver to be diagnosed with confidence on small biopsy samples; however, although there may be histological clues for a specific cause, it may be difficult to distinguish a cause for hepatitis by morphological means alone.

Specific infectious and toxic causes of acute hepatocellular necrosis and inflammation

Infectious canine hepatitis due to canine adenovirus 1 causes a multisystemic disease involving the liver, kidney, brain and other organs. In the liver, infection results in severe centrilobular to bridging necrosis with or without inflammation.

Amphophilic to basophilic intranuclear inclusion bodies are usually easily found in hepatocytes and may also occur in endothelial cells and bile duct epithelium (Figs 7.20, 7.21, 8.21).

Canine and feline herpes viruses cause a multisystemic disease involving the liver, kidneys, lungs and other organs. In the liver there are multifocal randomly dispersed areas of acute hepatocellular necrosis with or without inflammation (Fig. 7.22) and often extending into the portal and perivenular connective tissue. A few eosinophilic intranuclear

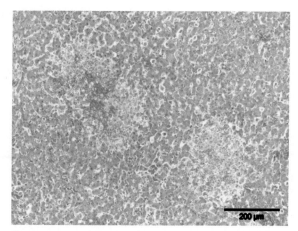

Figure 7.22 Canine herpes virus infection. Multifocal irregularly distributed coagulative necrosis. HE.

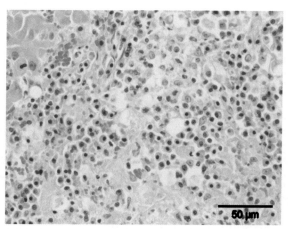

Figure 7.24 Feline infectious peritonitis virus infection. Focal fibrinoid necrosis and infiltration of macrophages and many plasma cells. HE.

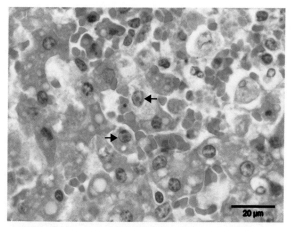

Figure 7.23 Canine herpes virus infection. Focal necrosis with intranuclear eosinophilic viral inclusions (arrows) in adjacent intact hepatocytes. HE.

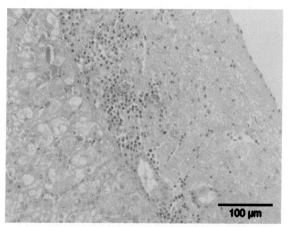

Figure 7.25 Feline infectious peritonitis virus infection. Liver covered by a thick layer of fibrin and a subcapsular mainly plasmacellular infiltrate. HE.

inclusion bodies with marginated nuclear chromatin may be seen in both hepatocytes and bile duct epithelium near or in the affected areas (Fig. 7.23).

Feline infectious peritonitis virus is a multisystemic disease involving the peritoneum, pleura, brain, eyes and parenchymal organs. In the liver there are frequently multifocal randomly dispersed areas of necrosis, often extending into the portal and perivenular connective tissue, with a moderate to marked infiltration of macrophages and, particularly at the periphery, plasma cells (Fig. 7.24); sometimes also fibrosis may be present. In cases of

peritoneal involvement the liver is covered by a thick layer of fibrin with some neutrophils and macrophages with infiltration of the liver capsule and subcapsular parenchyma by plasma cells and some lymphocytes (Fig. 7.25).

Clostridium piliformis (Tyzzer's disease) occurs in dogs and cats[7,8] and is characterized by randomly dispersed areas of confluent necrosis restricted to the parenchyma with or without an inflammatory reaction (Fig. 7.26). There are elongated large bacilli within viable hepatocytes at the margin of the necrotic foci. These can sometimes

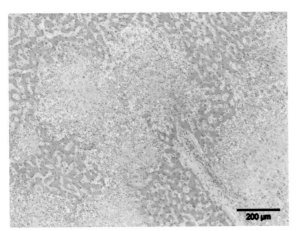

Figure 7.26   Tyzzer's disease. Multifocal necrosis restricted to the liver parenchyma. HE.

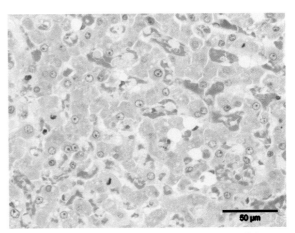

Figure 7.28   Leptospirosis. Slight dissociation of the liver cells and presence of many mitotic figures. HE.

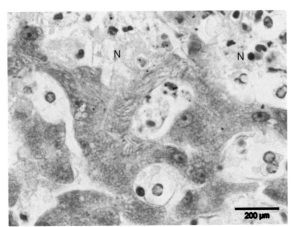

Figure 7.27   Tyzzer's disease. Viable hepatocytes with elongated large bacilli at the margin of the necrosis (N). Giemsa stain.

be seen in HE preparations, but are best seen with Giemsa or silver (Wartin-Starry) stains (Fig. 7.27).

Leptospirosis occurs in dogs and various serovars produce an acute multisystemic disease affecting the kidney, liver and other organs. Although large numbers of organisms are present in the liver, particularly in the space of Disse, hepatocellular necrosis usually is unremarkable or minimal, the main and characteristic lesion is dissociation and separation of liver cell plates (particularly evident in postmortem material) and the presence of many hepatocytes with mitotic figures or binucleation (Fig. 7.28). Moreover, slight sinusoidal and portal inflammation may be observed compatible with a non-specific reactive hepatitis (see Ch. 8).[9]

Helicobacter canis has been described in a young dog[10] and causes multifocal hepatic necrosis. The organisms were present at the periphery of the lesions and appeared to be located in bile canaliculi suggesting ascending infection along the bile ducts.

Septicemic bacterial diseases show a nonspecific reactive hepatitis (vide infra) and may be manifested by multifocal random focal and confluent necrosis with secondary Kupffer cell/macrophage proliferation and/or infiltration with neutrophilic leukocytes, and in a later stage lymphocytes and plasma cells. Many bacteria may cause hepatitis in dogs and cats, e.g. *Escherichia coli*, *Streptococcus*, *Pasteurella*, *Salmonella*, and *Brucella*. Bacterial culture and/or polymerase chain reaction (PCR) are necessary to identify the specific cause, but special stains (Gram, Warthin-Starry) may be helpful in determining or confirming the causative organism.

Toxoplasma gondii causes multisystemic disease involving the liver, lung, brain and other organs in the cat and dog. In the liver there is necrosis which may extend from focal to confluent areas of necrosis or in severe cases to panlobular involvement. Inflammation is usually seen and may include neutrophils, macrophages and other inflammatory cells. Areas of necrosis and the adjacent parenchyma often contain free tachyzoites and/or cysts containing bradyzoites (Fig. 7.29).[11,12]

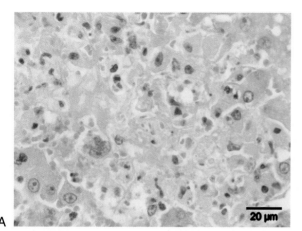

A

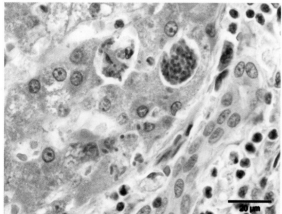

B

Figure 7.29   Toxoplasmosis. A Hepatic necrosis with many free tachyzoites. B pseudocyst. HE.

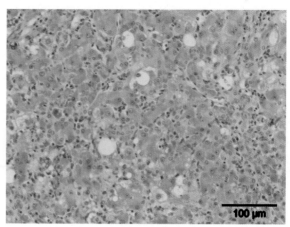

Figure 7.30   Dog. Chronic hepatitis with slight fibrosis, moderate inflammation, some apoptotic bodies and marked ductular proliferation. HE.

tion resulting in hepatic necrosis with or without inflammation.

Chronic hepatitis

General

Chronic hepatitis is characterized by hepatocellular apoptosis or necrosis, a variable mononuclear or mixed inflammatory infiltrate, regeneration and fibrosis (Figs 7.30, 7.31). The proportion and distribution of these components vary widely and it is necessary to include in the diagnosis the *activity and stage of the disease* as well as the possible etiology. The activity of the disease is determined by the quantity of inflammation and extent of hepatocellular apoptosis and necrosis which may be present as interface hepatitis and in a random focal or confluent pattern within the lobule. The stage of the disease, and thus the possible prognosis, is determined by the extent and pattern of fibrosis and the possible presence of architectural distortion (see cirrhosis). Fibrosis may present as porto-portal, porto-central and centro-central fibrosis or lobular dissecting. It may occur associated with interface hepatitis following collapse and condensation of the reticulin network or by direct activation of hepatic stellate cells with perisinusoidal deposition of collagen. Regeneration and regenerative nodules of hepatic parenchyma are often seen,

Amanitum spp, **a poisonous mushroom, intoxication** causes acute massive hepatic necrosis involving most of the liver (Fig. 7.12).

Cyanophyceae (blue green algae) intoxication with *Anabaena*, *Aphanizomenon* and *Microcystis* has been associated with massive hepatic necrosis in dogs.[13,14]

Benzodiazepine (Diazepam[R]) intoxication may cause an idiosyncratic drug reaction in cats associated with centrolobular, bridging and panlobular necrosis.[15]

Acetaminophen (paracetamol) has a direct dose-dependent toxic effect on the liver and may cause centrolobular, bridging and panlobular necrosis in both dogs and cats.[14]

Trimethoprim sulfonamide,[16] **carprofen,**[17] **and amiodarone**[18] may cause an idiosyncratic reac-

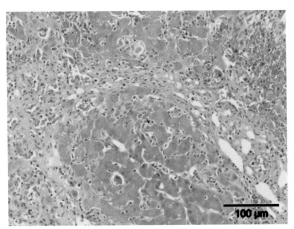

Figure 7.31 Dog. Chronic hepatitis with marked fibrosis and marked inflammation. HE.

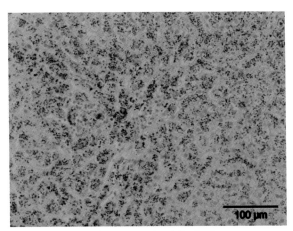

Figure 7.32 Bedlington terrier. Inherited copper toxicosis. Marked accumulation of copper in the hepatocytes and a mononuclear inflammatory infiltrate with some copper-containing macrophages. Rubeanic acid stain for copper.

as well as proliferation of ductular structures at the periphery of the parenchyma and within fibrous septa. Histochemical stains for connective tissue (reticulin stain according to Gordon and Sweet, Sirius red, Van Gieson's stain and trichrome stains) may be helpful in detecting the amount and pattern of fibrosis, particularly in early and mild disease.

The cause of most spontaneous cases of canine chronic hepatitis is undetermined although some cases have been associated with leptospirosis,[19] experimental and spontaneous infectious canine hepatitis virus infection.[20,21] Chronic hepatitis has also been reported in dogs treated with anticonvulsant drugs such as primidone, phenytoin, phenobarbital[22–24] and aflatoxicosis.[25,26] Chronic hepatitis and cirrhosis are rarely seen in cats.

Copper-associated chronic hepatitis

In the Bedlington terrier a genetic mutation in copper transport proteins causes accumulation of copper in hepatocytes resulting in inflammation or necrosis (Fig. 7.32).[27,28] Copper accumulation leading to inflammation and necrosis appears to be familial in the West Highland white terrier,[29] Skye terrier,[30] Dalmatian[31] and Labrador retriever,[32] and probably occurs in other breeds. In these animals, copper accumulates in hepatocytes, starting in the centrolobular regions, and with progressive accumulation, results in hepatocellular necrosis, inflam-

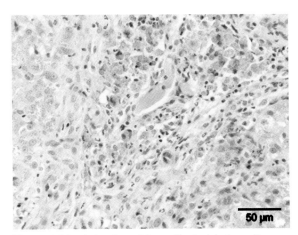

Figure 7.33 Labrador retriever. Centrolobular collapse and accumulation of copper- and ceroid-containing macrophages as well as copper-laden hepatocytes in the adjacent parenchyma. HE.

mation with copper-laden macrophages and finally chronic hepatitis and cirrhosis (Figs 7.33, 7.34).

Healthy dogs with normal livers may have copper levels up to 500 μg per g dry weight. Hepatic copper levels in breeds with primary copper storage disease vary between individual animals and between breeds. Bedlington terriers, West Highland white terriers, Dalmatians and Labrador retrievers with copper-associated liver

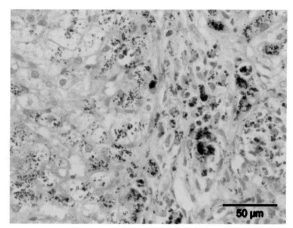

Figure 7.34   Labrador retriever. Centrolobular collaps with copper-laden macrophages and copper accumulation in the adjacent hepatocytes. Rubeanic acid stain for copper.

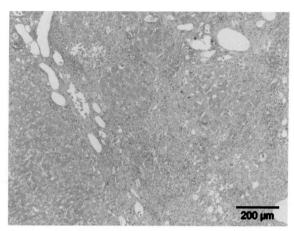

Figure 7.35   Dog. Cirrhosis. Broad bands of fibrous tissue with ductular proliferation and inflammation, vascular anastomoses, and regenerative nodules of varying size. HE.

damage reportedly have liver copper concentrations greater than 2000 µg per g of dry weight liver. Affected Skye terriers have concentrations ranging from 800–2200 µg per g. Other breeds (Doberman pinschers and American and English cocker spaniels) have been reported to have elevated copper concentrations in association with chronic hepatitis but it remains to be determined whether this copper accumulation is primary or secondary to chronic inflammation, fibrosis, and cholestasis or cholate-stasis.

Copper-induced chronic hepatitis and cirrhosis was recently observed in a cat and was characterized by severe copper deposition in hepatocytes and macrophages in the fibrotic areas and slight to moderate copper deposition in the regenerative nodules.[33]

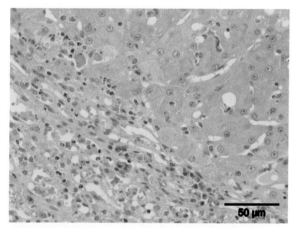

Figure 7.36   Dog. Cirrhosis. Newly formed fibrous septum with moderate inflammation and interface hepatitis. HE.

Cirrhosis

General

Cirrhosis is the end-stage of chronic hepatitis and is defined as a diffuse process characterized by fibrosis of the liver and the conversion of normal liver architecture into structurally abnormal nodules, and the presence of portal-central vascular anastomosis (Figs 7.35, 7.36).[34,35] As for chronic hepatitis it is essential to include in the diagnosis the extent of the fibrosis, the activity of

the disease and the possible etiology. Portal-portal fibrosis without other architectural changes does not constitute cirrhosis, but instead represents biliary-type fibrosis.

In cirrhosis, two morphological categories can be distinguished, i.e. **micronodular cirrhosis** with nodules less than 3 mm (the size of a normal lobule) that are all the same size (Fig. 7.37), and **macronodular cirrhosis** with nodules greater than 3 mm (up to several cm) (Figs 7.38, 7.39) that are of different sizes. Whereas micronodular cirrhosis

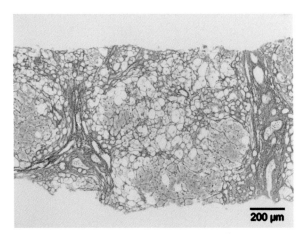

Figure 7.37   Dog. Micronodular cirrhosis. Gordon and Sweet stain for reticulin.

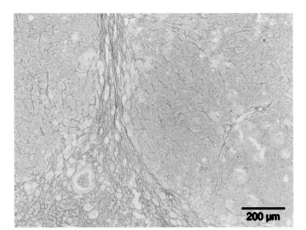

Figure 7.38   Dog. Macronodular cirrhosis. Gordon and Sweet stain for reticulin.

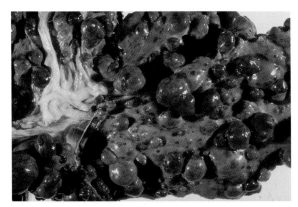

Figure 7.39   Dog. Macronodular cirrhosis.

develops from regular and diffuse alteration and fibrosis of the acini, macronodular cirrhosis develops from irregularly distributed larger areas of necrosis with secondary collapse and scarring and the development of portal-central vascular connections.[34,35]

Cirrhosis is a rather common condition in dogs and is often associated with portal hypertension and the presence of multiple portosystemic collateral veins. Some animals may have compensated cirrhotic disease and show no or minor clinical signs, while other animals show manifestations of liver failure, e.g. hyperbilirubinemia, coagulopathies, edema due to hypoalbuminemia, ascites and hepatoencephalopathy.

Cirrhosis is much less common in cats and diffuse hepatic fibrosis in cats usually represents porto-portal bridging fibrosis associated with chronic biliary disease.

Lobular dissecting hepatitis

Lobular dissecting hepatitis is a form of cirrhosis seen in premature and young adult dogs as isolated cases or in groups of dogs from the same litter or kennel, and it has a rapid clinical course.[36] The liver usually is of normal size with a smooth capsular surface or some small nodules of regeneration (Fig. 7.40). Microscopically, bands of fibroblasts

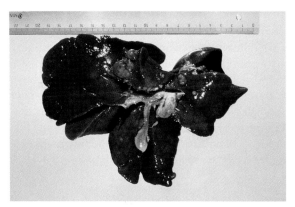

Figure 7.40   Dog. Lobular dissecting hepatitis. (Reproduced from van den Ingh TSGAM, Rothuizen J. Lobular dissecting hepatitis in juvenile and young adult dogs. J Vet Intern Med 1994; 8:217–220, with permission).

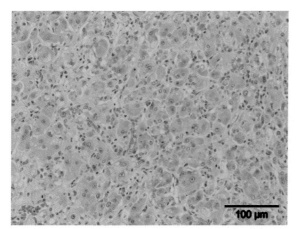

Figure 7.41   Dog. Lobular dissecting hepatitis. HE.

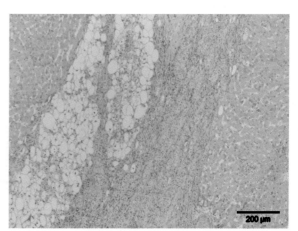

Figure 7.43   Dog. Cirrhosis in superficial necrolytic dermatitis characterized by large hyperplastic regenerative nodules separated by a band of fibrous tissue with ductular proliferation and slight inflammation, and areas of clear ballooned hepatocytes at the border of the nodules. HE.

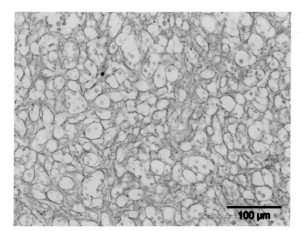

Figure 7.42   Lobular dissecting hepatitis. Gordon and Sweet stain for reticulin.

atic tumors.[37-39] The skin lesion is characterized by basal cell hyperplasia, edema of the stratum spinosum and parakeratotic hyperkeratosis. The livers in this disease are strikingly similar and show a peculiar form of macronodular cirrhosis. They are divided into regenerative hyperplastic nodules by fibrous septa containing ductular structures and pigment-laden macrophages, and show minimal or no inflammation and hepatocellular necrosis. The nodules are characteristically bordered by areas of clear ballooned hepatocytes similar to steroid-induced hepatopathy (Fig. 7.43). The nodules show minimal or no inflammation and necrosis.

Non-specific reactive hepatitis

Non-specific reactive hepatitis is a morphological entity widespread within the liver. It represents a non-specific response to a variety of extrahepatic disease processes, especially febrile illnesses and inflammation somewhere in the splanchnic bed, or it represents the residual lesion of a previous inflammatory intrahepatic disease.[40] The lesion is characterized by an inflammatory infiltrate in portal areas and in the parenchyma without evident hepatocellular necrosis. In acute extrahepatic diseases there is a slight to moderate infiltrate of mainly neutrophils in the stroma of the portal areas

and thin strands of extracellular matrix are seen between individual and small groups of hepatocytes, which cause dissection of the original lobular architecture (Fig. 7.41). Connective tissue stains (especially for reticulin) are helpful in demonstrating the pattern of connective tissue alterations (Fig. 7.42). Inflammation and hepatocellular apoptosis/necrosis are usually slight to moderate.

Cirrhosis in superficial necrolytic dermatitis

Superficial necrolytic dermatitis (hepatocutaneous syndrome) is a cutaneous disease in dogs usually associated with chronic hepatic disorders and rarely glucagon-producing endocrine pancre-

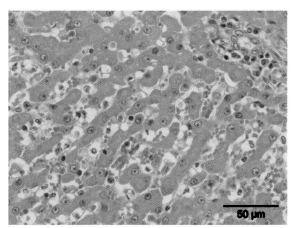

Figure 7.44 Dog. Non-specific reactive hepatitis. Kupffer cell proliferation and (degenerated) neutrophils in the sinusoids and a mainly lympho-plasmacellular infiltrate in the portal area. HE.

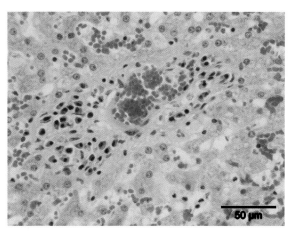

Figure 7.45 Dog. Non-specific reactive hepatitis. Plasmacellular infiltrate around the hepatic vein. HE.

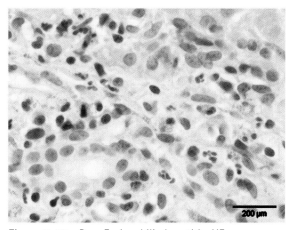

Figure 7.46 Dog. Eosinophilic hepatitis. HE.

that varies in intensity between portal areas and that may include normal portal areas. There is slight to marked leukocytosis and Kupffer cell proliferation in the sinusoids and some neutrophils in the stroma around the hepatic veins. In chronic extrahepatic diseases, or in the case of residual intrahepatic disease, the inflammation is usually mainly mononuclear with plasma cells and lymphocytes (and pigmented macrophages) in the portal areas and around the hepatic veins, as well as some plasma cells and lymphocytes with or without single or small aggregates of pigment-laden macrophages within the parenchyma (Figs 7.44, 7.45).

Eosinophilic hepatitis

Eosinophils appear mostly as scattered elements in portal and perivenous infiltrates and less frequently within the sinusoids, and can be observed in dogs and, probably more often, in cats (Fig. 7.46). They can be regarded as a non-specific reactive hepatitis particularly associated with allergic conditions and hypereosinophilic syndromes. Marked eosinophilic inflammation in the liver is a rare condition in dogs and cats and may be associated with parasitic infections (migrating nematode larvae, schistosomiasis, liver fluke infestation) usually at and near the site of the parasitic lesion; a more diffuse lesion is sometimes seen in drug-induced liver lesions, e.g. trimethropim/sulpha (TMPS).

SUMMARY

This chapter presents the various forms of hepatocellular death: apoptosis and necrosis, the morphological patterns of necrosis in the liver, and the response of the liver to hepatocellular injury. The definition and characteristics of acute and chronic hepatitis and cirrhosis are given, including copper-associated chronic hepatitis, lobular dissecting hepatitis and cirrhosis associated with superficial necrolytic dermatitis. Moreover, examples of specific infectious and non-infectious causes of hepatocellular necrosis and hepatitis are given.

Finally, the lesions and clinical significance of non-specific reactive hepatitis and eosinophilic hepatitis are presented.

References

1. Cotran RS, Kumar V, Collins T. Robbins: pathologic basis of disease. Philadelphia: WB Saunders; 2000.
2. Zeiss CJ. The apoptosis-necrosis continuum: insight from genetically altered mice. Vet Pathol 2003; 40:481–495.
3. Patel T. Apoptosis in hepatic pathophysiology. Clinics in Liver Disease 2000; 4:295–317.
4. Ferrell LD, Theise ND, Scheuer PJ. Acute and chronic viral hepatitis. In: McSween RNM, Burt AD, Portmann BC, et al, eds. Pathology of the liver. 4th edn. Edinburgh: Churchill Livingstone; 2002:313–362.
5. Poulsen H, Christoffersen P. Atlas of liver biopsies. 1st edn. Copenhagen: Munksgaard; 1979.
6. Kelly WR. The liver and biliary system. In: Jubb KVF, Kennedy PC, Palmer N, eds. Pathology of domestic animals. 4th edn. San Diego: Academic Press; 1992:319–406.
7. Qureshi SR, Carlton WW, Olander HJ. Tyzzer's disease in a dog. J Am Vet Med Assoc 1976; 168(7):602–604.
8. Kubokawa K, Kubo M, Takasaki Y, et al. Two cases of feline Tyzzer's disease. Jpn J Exp Med 1973; 43(5):413–421.
9. Hartman EG, Van den Ingh TSGAM, Rothuizen J. Clinical, pathological and serological features of spontaneous canine leptospirosis: An evaluation of the IgM and IgG specific Elisa. Vet Immunol Immunopathol 1986; 13:261–271.
10. Fox JG, Drolet R, Higgins R, et al. Helicobacter canis isolated from a dog liver with multifocal necrotizing hepatitis. J Clin Microbiol 1996; 34:2479–2482.
11. Dubey JP, Zajac A, Osofsky SA, et al. Acute primary toxoplasmic hepatitis in an adult cat shedding Toxoplasma gondii oocysts. J Am Vet Med Assoc 1990; 197(12):1616–1618.
12. Dubey JP, Mattix ME, Lipscomb TP. Lesions of neonatally induced toxoplasmosis in cats. Vet Pathol 1996; 33(3):290–295.
13. DeVries SE, Galey FD, Namikoshi M, et al. Clinical and pathologic findings of blue-green algae (Microcystis aeruginosa) intoxication in a dog. J Vet Diagn Invest 1993; 5(3):403–408.
14. Cullen JM, MacLachlan NJ. Liver, biliary system and pancreas. In: McGavin MD, Carlton WW, Zachary JF, eds. Thomson's special veterinary pathology. 3rd

edn. Mosby: Press: St Louis; 2001: 81–123.
15. Center SA, Elston TH, Rowland PH, et al. Fulminant hepatic failure associated with oral administration of diazepam in 11 cats. J Am Vet Med Assoc 1996; 209(3):618–625.
16. Twedt DC, Diehl KJ, Lappin MR, et al. Association of hepatic necrosis with trimethoprim sulfonamide administration in 4 dogs. J Vet Intern Med 1997; 11(1):20–23.
17. MacPhail CM, Lappin MR, Meyer DJ, et al. Hepatocellular toxicosis associated with administration of carprofen in 21 dogs. J Am Vet Med Assoc 1998; 212(12):1895–1901.
18. Jacobs G, Calvert C, Kraus M. Hepatopathy in 4 dogs treated with amiodarone. J Vet Intern Med 2000; 14(1):96–99.
19. Adamus C, Buggin-Daubie M, Izembart A, et al. Chronic hepatitis associated with leptospiral infection in vaccinated beagles. J Comp Pathol 1997; 117(4):311–328.
20. Gocke DJ, Preisig R, Morris TQ, et al. Experimental viral hepatitis in the dog: production and persistent disease in partially immune animals. J Clin Investigations 1967; 46:1505–1517.
21. Rakich PM, Prasse KW, Lukert PD, et al. Immunohistochemical detection of canine adenovirus in paraffin sections of liver. Vet Pathol 1986; 23:478–484.
22. Bunch SE, Castleman WL, Hornbuckle WE, et al. Hepatic cirrhosis associated with long-term anticonvulsant drug therapy in dogs. J Am Vet Med Assoc 1982; 181(4):357–362.
23. Dayrell-Hart B, Steinberg SA, Van Winkle TJ, et al. Hepatotoxicity of phenobarbital in dogs: 18 cases (1985–1989). J Am Vet Med Assoc 1991; 199:1060–1066.
24. Poffenbarger EM, Hardy RM. Hepatic cirrhosis associated with long-term primidone therapy in a dog. J Am Vet Med Assoc 1985; 186(9): 978–980.
25. Newberne PM. Chronic aflatoxicosis. J Am Vet Med Assoc 1973; 163(11):1262–1267.
26. Chaffee VW, Edds GT, Himes JA, et al. Aflatoxicosis in dogs. Am J Vet Res 1969; 30(10):1737–1749.
27. van De Sluis B, Rothuizen J, Pearson PL, et al. Identification of a new copper metabolism gene by

positional cloning in a purebred dog population. Hum Mol Genet 2002; 11(2):165–173.

28. Twedt DC, Sternlieb I, Gilbertson SR. Clinical, morphologic, and chemical studies on copper toxicosis of Bedlington Terriers. J Am Vet Med Assoc 1979; 175(3):269–275.

29. Thornburg LP, Shaw D, Dolan M, et al. Hereditary copper toxicosis in West Highland white terriers. Vet Pathol 1986; 23(2):148–154.

30. Haywood S, Rutgers HC, Christian MK. Hepatitis and copper accumulation in Skye terriers. Vet Pathol 1988; 25:408–414.

31. Webb CB, Twedt DC, Meyer DJ. Copper-associated liver disease in Dalmatians: a review of 10 dogs (1998–2001). J Vet Intern Med 2002; 16(6):665–668.

32. Hoffman G, Van den Ingh TSGAM, Rothuizen J. Copper-associated hepatitis in Labrador retrievers: 15 clinical cases and their family (1999–2002). In: 23rd ACVIM Forum; 2005; Baltimore, USA; 2005.

33. Meertens NM, Bokhove CA, Van den Ingh TS. Copper-associated chronic hepatitis and cirrhosis in a European shorthair cat. Vet Pathol 2005; 42(1):97–100.

34. Anthony HD, Ishak KG, Nayak NC, et al. The morphology of cirrhosis: Definition, nomenclature and classification. Bull WHO 1977; 55:521–540.

35. Crawford JM. Liver cirrhosis. In: McSween RNM, Burt AD, Portmann BC, eds. Pathology of the liver. 4th edn. Edinburgh: Churchill Livingstone; 2002:575–620.

36. van den Ingh TSGAM, Rothuizen J. Lobular dissecting hepatitis in juvenile and young adult dogs. J Vet Intern Med 1994; 8:217–220.

37. Gross TL, Song MD, Havel PJ, et al. Superficial necrolytic dermatitis (necrolytic migratory erythema) in dogs. Vet Pathol 1993; 30(1):75–81.

38. Gross TL, O'Brien TD, Davies AP, et al. Glucagon-producing pancreatic endocrine tumors in two dogs with superficial necrolytic dermatitis. J Am Vet Med Assoc 1990; 197(12):1619–1622.

39. March PA, Hillier A, Weisbrode SE, et al. Superficial necrolytic dermatitis in 11 dogs with a history of phenobarbital administration (1995–2002). J Vet Intern Med 2004; 18:65–74.

40. Burt AD, Portmann BC, McSween RNM. Liver pathology associated with diseases of other organs or systems. In: McSween RNM, Burt AD, Portmann BC, eds. Pathology of the liver. 4th edn. Edinburgh: Churchill Livingstone; 2002.

Chapter 8

Morphological classification of parenchymal disorders of the canine and feline liver

3. Hepatic abcesses and granulomas, hepatic metabolic storage disorders and miscellaneous conditions

Tom Van Winkle, John M. Cullen, Ted S. G. A. M. van den Ingh, Jenny A. Charles, Valeer J. Desmet

HEPATIC ABSCESSES AND GRANULOMAS

Hepatic abscesses are usually the result of bacterial infections that lead to intense accumulation and subsequent lysis of neutrophilic granulocytes at the infection site (Fig. 8.1). They can reach the liver via different routes including the portal vein or umbilical vein, ascending infection of the biliary system, and by direct contact and penetration of the liver capsule. Hepatic abscesses in dogs and cats are particularly seen in newborn animals due to umbilical infection (e.g. several Gram-positive and Gram-negative bacteria). In adult animals, hepatic abscesses are often the result of infections with *Yersinia* spp. (Fig. 8.2), *Nocardia asteroides* and *Actinomyces* spp.[1,2] Hepatic abscesses may occur in association with central necrosis of hepatocellular neoplasms.

Hepatic granulomas may occur in a wide variety of diseases, some of which are primary in the liver, but most are part of a generalized disease process. They consist of (multi)focal aggregations of activated macrophages with an epithelioid appearance, mostly infiltrated by lymphocytes and plasma cells and possibly fibroblasts, and may be

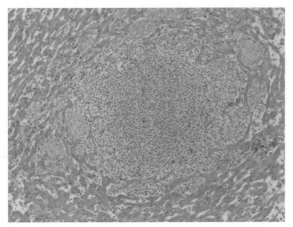

Figure 8.1   Dog. Hepatic abscess with fibrinoid deposits at the periphery. HE.

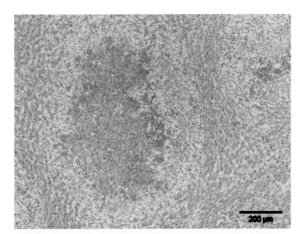

Figure 8.2   Cat. Hepatic abscess due to *Yersinia* with centrally located bacteria. HE.

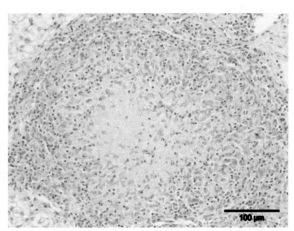

Figure 8.3   Dog. Tubercle with epithelioid cells, central caseous necrosis and peripheral lymphocytic infiltrate. Note absence of Langhans type multinucleated giant cells. Mycobacterium tuberculosis. HE.

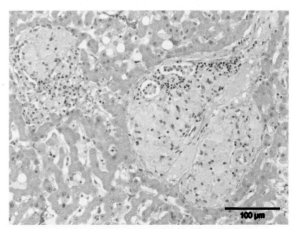

Figure 8.4   Cat. Epithelioid granulomas in the portal area and parenchyma. Mycobacterium avium. HE.

surrounded by collagen fibers. Epithelioid cells may fuse to form multinucleated giant cells; the nuclei may either be arranged peripherally (Langhans-type giant cell) or haphazardly (foreign-body-type giant cell).[3] The classic example of granulomatous disease is tuberculosis. The granulomas, referred to as tubercles, are characterized by the presence of epithelioid cells and Langhans-type giant cells with central caseous necrosis and a peripheral zone of lymphocytes (Fig. 8.3); in contrast to other domestic animal species, giant cells of the Langhans type are only rarely observed in both dogs and cats.[4]

Infectious causes for hepatic granulomas in dogs and cats include mycobacterial infections (*M.* *tuberculosis* (Fig. 8.3), *M. avium intracellulare* (Figs 8.4, 8.5)), systemic mycoses (*Blastomyces dermatitidis, Cryptococcus neoformans, Histoplasma capsulatum, Coccidioides immitis*) and opportunistic fungal infections (Fig. 8.6), migrating nematode larvae (visceral larva migrans) and schistosomiasis. A diffuse granulomatous inflammation of the liver is observed in *Leishmania* infection (Fig. 8.7) in dogs[5] and *Cytauxzoon felis* infection (Fig. 8.8) in cats;[6] in both cases large numbers of amastigotes respectively schizonts may

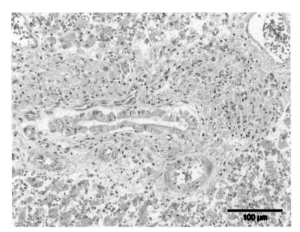

Figure 8.5 Dog. Epithelioid granulomatous inflammation in the portal area. Mycobacterium avium. HE.

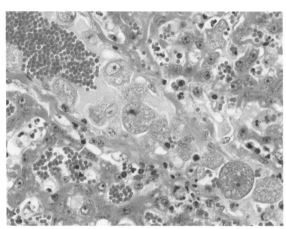

Figure 8.8 Cat. Cytauxoon felis infection. Large numbers of schizonts in Kupffer cells and macrophages. HE.

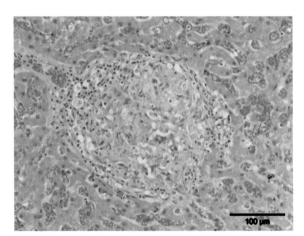

Figure 8.6 Dog. Mycotic granuloma. HE.

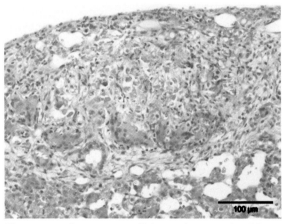

Figure 8.9 Dog, neonate. Subcapsular necrosis with dystrophic calcification and subsequent granulomatous inflammation. HE.

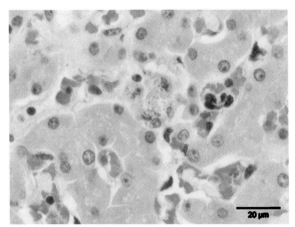

Figure 8.7 Dog. Leishmaniasis. Amastigotes in the cytoplasm of Kupffer cells/macrophages. HE.

be observed in Kupffer cells and macrophages. Granulomatous and non-suppurative hepatitis has been reported in the dog in association with *Bartonella* spp.[7]

Granulomas may also be incited by relatively inert foreign material (e.g. crystalline material, sutures, plant material). In neonates, subcapsular hepatocellular necrosis (probably associated with asphyxia) with subsequent mineralization and granulomatous inflammation may be seen at the periphery of the liver lobes (Fig. 8.9).

HEPATIC METABOLIC STORAGE DISORDERS

General

Hepatic metabolic storage disorders, usually associated with inherited but sometimes acquired metabolic enzyme deficiencies, can have a variety of morphological appearances (Table 8.1). The most common finding is the presence of clear vacuoles, vacuoles with granular or hyaline material, or pigmented granules in hepatocytes and/or Kupffer cells and macrophages (Figs 8.10, 8.11). Rarely, as in glycogenosis type I and III, the lesion is characterized by markedly swollen, clear hepatocytes with well-outlined cell membranes giving the hepatocytes the appearance of plant cells.

These changes are usually non-specific and can be better evaluated in frozen or plastic-embedded sections using conventional, lectin- and immuno-histochemistry or electron microscopy. However, diagnosis depends on either the identification of the storage product or the enzyme deficiency by biochemical methods, or by identification of the genetic defect. Although the changes may be insufficient to cause hepatocellular or Kupffer cell necrosis, particularly severe hepatocellular storage may result in hepatocellular necrosis and inflammation, and even chronic hepatitis and cirrhosis may develop.

Erythropoietic protoporphyria

Erythropoietic protoporphyria is known in dogs as an acquired storage disease following administration of a number of xenobiotics, e.g. griseofulvin and the antiarthritic drug 3-[2-(2,4,6-trimethylphenyl)-thiothyl]methylsydnoneis (TTMS).[8] Drug-induced protoporphyria is a result of inhibition of ferrochelatase, compensatory stimulation of the first enzyme in the 5-aminolevulate synthase pathway and massive accumulation of the substrate protoporphyrin. Protoporphyrin is recognized as dark brown pigment in canaliculi and interlobular bile ducts, and in more severe cases also in Kupffer cells and macrophages (Fig. 8.12). The pigment displays bright red birefringence with a centrally located dark Maltese cross. Occasionally severe deposition of the pigment may result in chronic hepatitis and cirrhosis.[9,10]

MISCELLANEOUS CONDITIONS

Hepatocytes

Cytoplasmic alterations

- **Protein droplets** are variably sized eosinophilic (hyaline) droplets in the cytoplasm of hepatocytes (Fig. 8.13). They may consist of engulfed serum proteins and represent a non-specific and variable finding associated with shock, ischemia, or other acute hepatocellular injury. They may also consist of fibrinogen and acute phase proteins (alpha-1-antitrypsin, haptoglobin, alpha-macroglobulin) retained in the endoplasmic reticulum in hepatocytes as seen in dogs with chronic hepatitis and cirrhosis.[11]
- **Eosinophilic cytoplasmic bodies** of variable size may be the result of phagocytosis of apoptotic bodies by hepatocytes.
- **'Ground glass' appearance:** swollen hepatocytes with pink finely granular to hyaline cytoplasm (Fig. 8.14). These changes are associated with an increase in the smooth endoplasmic reticulum and induction of the hepatic microsomal drug metabolizing enzymes. The ground glass appearance of the hepatocytes may be caused by drugs (e.g. phenobarbital) and other substances that cause induction of cytochrome P450 enzymes.
- **Lipofuscin:** this is brown-yellow pigmented granular material in hepatocytes within lysosomes and is most abundant in a pericanalicular location (Fig. 8.15). It is present in normal livers in varying amounts. Increased hepatocellular lipofuscin occurs with age, particularly in cats, and is most prominent in the centrilobular hepatocytes.
- **Accumulation of copper** is seen as gray-yellow to gray-brown or gray-blue granules in the cytoplasm. The color of the granules may vary depending on tissue preparation procedures used by the laboratory (Fig. 8.16). Copper can be specifically identified by histochemical stains (e.g. rubeanic acid or rhodanine for copper and orcein for copper-binding protein). Storage of copper can be primary due to a genetic defect in one of the genes associated with copper metabolism, such as in inherited copper toxicosis in Bedlington terriers, or secondary to

Table 8.1   Hepatic metabolic storage disorders

Disease name	Stored material	Defective enzyme	Morphology of stored material	Hepatocytes	Kupffer cells/ macrophages	Species/breed
Ceroid-lipofuscinosis	Ceroid/lipofuscin	Unknown	Granules (yellow-brown)		X	Canine[15-17] Feline[17,18]
Cholesterol ester storage disease	Cholesterol esters and cholesterol in Kupffer cells and macrophages; neutral lipids and cholesterol in hepatocytes	Acid lipase Fox terrier[19]	Clear vacuoles and cholesterol crystals	X	X	Canine
Fucosidosis	Fucose containing glycolipids, glycoproteins, poly-/ oligo-saccharides	Alpha-L-fucosidase	Clear vacuoles		X	Canine[20,21] English springer spaniel
Galactosialidosis	Glycolipids and oligosaccharides	Beta galactosidase, alpha-neuraminidase	Clear vacuoles	X	X	Canine[22] Schipperke dog
GM 1 gangliosidosis	Gangliosides	Beta-galactosidase	Clear vacuoles	X	X	Canine[22-28] Portugese waterdogs, Shiba dogs, Alaskan Huskies, English springer spaniel, mixed breed dog Feline[29,30] Siamese, Korat
GM2 gangliosidosis	Gangliosides	Beta-hexosaminidase A/B	Clear vacuoles	X	X	Canine[31-33] Japanese spaniel, German short-haired pointer, Golden retriever, Feline[34] DSH[a]
Glycogenosis type IA	Glycogen	Glucose-6-phosphatase	Swollen clear cells		X	Canine[35] Maltese dog
Glycogenosis type III	Glycogen	Amylo-1,6-glucosidase	Swollen clear cells	X		Canine[36,37] German shepherd dog
Glycogenosis type IV	Abnormally branched glycogen (alpha-1,4-D-glucan)	Branching enzyme	Pale blue granules	X	X	Feline[38] Norwegian forest cat

Table 8.1 Hepatic metabolic storage disorders—(continued)

Disease name	Stored material	Defective enzyme	Morphology of stored material	Hepatocytes	Kupffer cells/ macrophages	Species/breed
Glycosyl ceramide lipidosis (Gaucher's disease)	Glycosyl ceramines	Acid beta-glucosidase	Pale, faintly striated inclusions		X	Canine[39,40] Silky terrier
Inherited copper toxicosis	Copper	Unknown	Granules (blue-grey, yellow-brown, red-brown)	X	X (secondary)	Canine (see Ch.8 for copper-associated chronic hepatitis)
Mannosidosis	Glycoprotein derived mannose-rich oligosaccharides	Alpha or beta mannosidase	Clear vacuoles	X	X	Feline[41–43] Persian, DSH, DLH[b]
Mucolipidosis type II	Mucopolysaccharids, lipids, glycoproteins	N-acetyl glucosamine-1-phosphotransferase	Clear vacuoles		X (Fibroblasts/endothelial lining cells)	Feline[44] DSH
Mucopolysaccharidosis type I	Heparan and dermatan sulphate	Alpha-L-iduronidase	Clear vacuoles	X	X	Canine[45,46] Plott hound Feline[45,47] DSH
Mucopolysaccharidosis type II	Heparan and dermatan sulphate	Alpha-L-iduronidase sulphatase	Clear vacuoles	X	X	Canine[48] Labrador retriever
Mucopolysaccharidosis type III	Heparan sulphate	Heparan sulphatase	Clear vacuoles	X	X	Canine[49–51] Wirehaired Dachshund, New Zealand Huntaway
Mucopolysaccharidosis type VI	Dermatan sulphate	Arylsulphatase B	Clear vacuoles	X	X	Canine[16,52] Miniature Schnauzer, Miniature Pinscher Feline[16,45,53] DSH, Siamese
Mucopolysaccharidosis type VII	Chondroitin and dermatan sulphate	Beta-glucuronidase	Clear vacuoles	X	X	Canine[45,54] Mixed breed Feline[55,56] DSH
Primary hyperlipoproteinaemia	Lipids	Lipoprotein lipase	Clear vacuoles	X	X (including xanthomata)	Feline[57,58]
Sphingomyelin-cholesterol lipidosis (Niemann-Pick disease type C)	Unesterified cholesterol	Acidic sphingomyelinase	Clear vacuoles		X	Canine[59,60] Miniature poodle, boxer Feline[61,62] DSH, Siamese

[a] DSH – domestic short hair; [b] DLH – domestic long hair

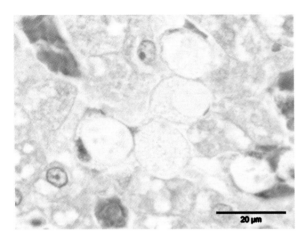

Figure 8.10   Dog. Fucosidosis. Swollen Kupffer cells – macrophages with vacuolization of the cytoplasm. HE.

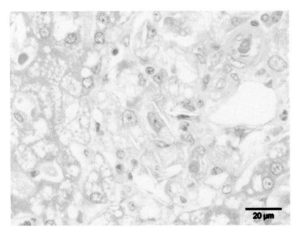

Figure 8.11   Dog. Cholesterol ester storage disease (Wolman's disease). Vacuolation of hepatocytes and vacuolation and cholesterol crystals in macrophages in the portal area. HE.

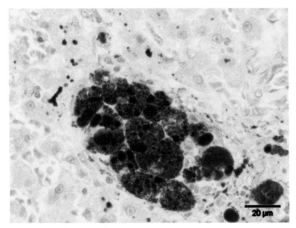

Figure 8.12   Dog. Erythropoietic protoporphyria. Dark brown pigment I (protoporphyrin) in canaliculi and in macrophages. HE.

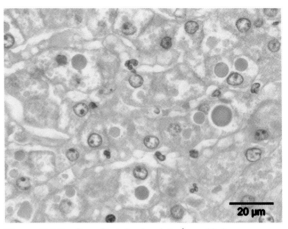

Figure 8.13   Dog. Protein droplets (engulfed serum proteins) in the hepatocytic cytoplasm. HE.

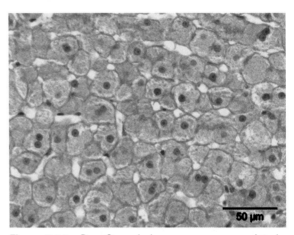

Figure 8.14   Dog. Ground glass appearance associated with phenobarbital medication. HE.

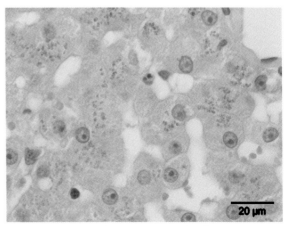

Figure 8.15   Cat. Lipofuscin deposition in a pericanalicular location in centrolobular hepatocytes. HE.

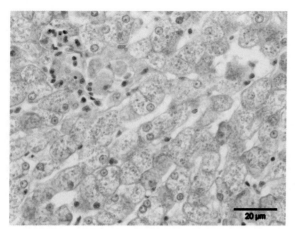

Figure 8.16 Bedlington terrier. Gray-yellow copper-containing granules diffusely dispersed in the hepatocytic cytoplasm. Inherited copper toxicosis. HE.

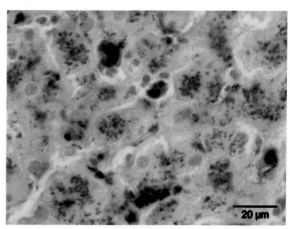

Figure 8.18 Cat (same animal as in Fig. 8.17). Blue staining iron pigment in hepatocytes and Kupffer cells. Prussian blue stain for iron.

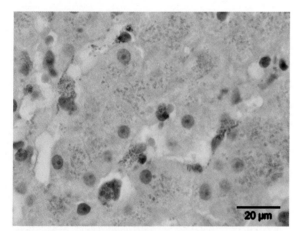

Figure 8.17 Cat. Brown iron-containing granules in the cytoplasm of hepatocytes and Kupffer cells. Erythremic myelosis. HE.

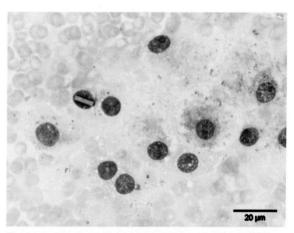

Figure 8.19 Dog. Cytological specimen. Intranuclear brick inclusion. May-Grünwald Giemsa stain.

cholestasis such as in chronic hepatitis and extra-hepatic bile duct obstruction.

- **Accumulation of iron** is seen as brown granules in the cytoplasm of hepatocytes (Figs 8.17, 8.18) and may be seen with increased red blood cell turnover, anemia of chronic disease and after administration of iron.
- **Emperipolesis** is a rare phenomenon of invagination of the cell membrane and engulfement of complete cells. It is particularly seen in epitheliotropic T-cell malignant lymphomas (see Fig. 9.20), where the neoplastic lymphocytes are engulfed by the hepatocytes.[12]

Nuclear alterations

- **'Brick' inclusions** (Fig. 8.19) are rectangular to rhomboid brightly eosinophilic bodies in the nuclei of hepatocytes in dogs, and are of no known significance.
- **Cytoplasmic invaginations** occur as round to oval protrusions of the cytoplasm into the nucleus and are of no known significance.
- **Glycogen inclusions** (Fig. 8.20) occur as clear inclusions in the nucleus and are of unknown significance. They are non-specific and may occur, e.g. in diabetes mellitus and hepatocellular neoplasia.

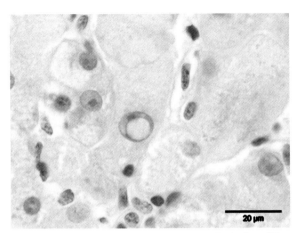

Figure 8.20   Dog. Intranuclear glycogen inclusion. HE.

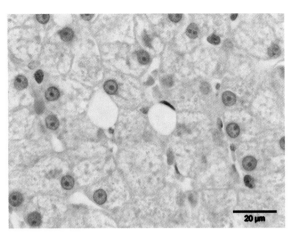

Figure 8.22   Dog. Hepatic stellate cell with a large lipid vacuole and displacement of the nucleus to the periphery of the cell. HE.

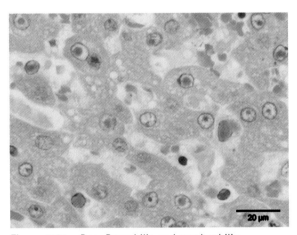

Figure 8.21   Dog. Basophilic and amphophilic intranuclear viral inclusions in hepatocytes and endothelial cells. Adenovirus type 1 infection. HE.

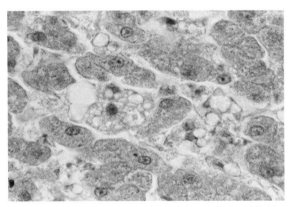

Figure 8.23   Cat. Hypertrophy and hyperplasia of lipid laden hepatic stellate cells. Vitamin A intoxication. HE. (Reproduced from Mouwen JMVM, De Groot ECBM, eds. Atlas of veterinary pathology. Utrecht: Bunge; 1982, with permission).

- **Intranuclear viral inclusions** (Fig. 8.21) may be observed in various viral infections (see different infectious causes of hepatitis in Ch. 7).
- **Intranuclear acid-fast inclusions** have been reported in dogs with lead intoxication but are extremely rare.[13]

Hepatic stellate cells

Hepatic stellate cells have large lipid vacuoles. Increased numbers of hepatic stellate cells are observed in older cats and are less pronounced in old dogs. They are recognized as solitary cells with a single large empty vacuole with displacement of the nucleus to the periphery of the cell (Fig. 8.22). The significance of this change is not known.

Chronic vitamin A intoxication is known in cats and causes hypertrophy and hyperplasia of lipid laden hepatic stellate cells (Fig. 8.23) as well as sinusoidal fibrosis with or without mild hepatocellular steatosis.

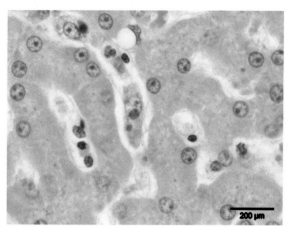

Figure 8.24   Dog. Erythrophagocytosis and hemosiderosis of Kupffer cell. Immune-mediated hemolytic anemia. HE.

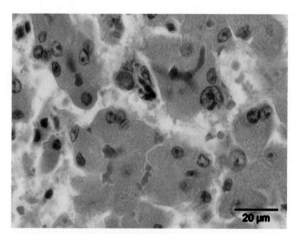

Figure 8.25   Dog. Bile plugs in canaliculi and phagocytosed bile plugs in Kupffer cells. HE.

Kuppfer cells

- **Necrosis** of Kupffer cells may be seen in sepsis and toxemia.
- **Erythrophagocytosis/hemosiderosis**   (Fig. 8.24) is observed in conditions with increased red cell turnover, such as hemolytic anemia, anemia of chronic disease and chronic hepatitis. The Kupffer cells may contain erythrocytes (erythrophagocytosis) and/or increased amounts of iron pigment (hemosiderosis).
- **Bile pigment** (Fig. 8.25) can be seen in cases with marked cholestasis and will be present as yellow-brown to yellow-green intracytoplasmic granules or bile plugs.

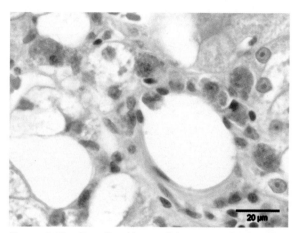

Figure 8.26   Dog. Ceroid containing macrophages. HE.

- **Eosinophilic cytoplasmic bodies** of variable size may be the result of phagocytosis of fragments of apoptotic cells by Kupffer cells.
- **Ceroid** is a yellow-brown, periodic acid Schiff (PAS) positive, lipid breakdown product that accumulates in Kupffer cells and macrophages as a result of increased hepatocyte turnover due to necrosis/apoptosis (Fig. 8.26).

Lipogranulomas (also known as fatty cysts[14]) and pigment granulomas

Lipogranulomas and pigment granulomas are poorly defined lesions of undetermined significance with overlapping features. **Lipogranulomas** are aggregates of ceroid-laden foamy fat-containing macrophages and sometimes also some lymphocytes and plasma cells (Fig. 8.27). They are probably associated with previous hepatocyte death and occur both in the parenchyma as well as in the portal and perivenular connective tissue. **Pigment granulomas** generally consist of both ceroid- and iron pigment containing macrophages (Fig. 8.28); lymphocytes or plasma cells are often also present. They are present throughout the parenchyma and are regularly seen, particularly in older animals, and have no known significance.

Extramedullary hemopoiesis

In both canine and feline neonates **extramedullary hemopoiesis** of all hematopoietic elements is a

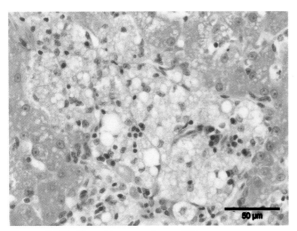

Figure 8.27   Dog. Lipogranuloma. HE.

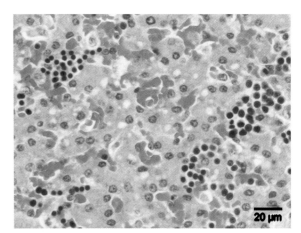

Figure 8.29   Dog, neonate. Extramedullary erythropoiesis. HE.

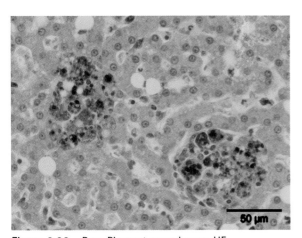

Figure 8.28   Dog. Pigment granulomas. HE.

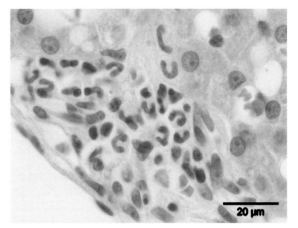

Figure 8.30   Dog. Extramedullary myelopoiesis. HE.

such as pyometra, and pleuritis or peritonitis due to nocardiosis or actinomycosis.

SUMMARY

Hepatic abscesses and granulomas usually occur by hematogenic spread from the portal vein or in neonates from the umbilical vein, and a wide variety of causative organisms are given. The various hepatic metabolic storage diseases in dogs and cats mentioned in the literature are summarized, including the enzymatic defect, the hepatic cells involved and their morphological aspect. Finally, miscellaneous conditions are presented which include cytoplasmic and nuclear alterations in hepatocytes, Kupffer cells and hepatic stellate cells as well as extramedullary hemopoiesis.

normal condition. Whereas the erythropoietic activity (Fig 8.29) and megakaryocytes are particularly seen in the parenchyma, the myelopoiesis is mainly seen in the stromal tissue of the portal and perivenular areas. In septicemic bacterial diseases the myelopoietic activity may be markedly increased.

In older dogs and less frequently in cats, **extramedullary erythropoiesis and megakaryocytes** can be observed in immune-mediated hemolytic anemia and thrombocytopenia. **Extramedullary myelopoiesis** (Fig 8.30) is regularly seen as small foci of band and segmented neutrophils in dogs with steroid-induced hepatopathy, and in chronic purulent inflammation

References

1. Farrar ET, Washabau RJ, Saunders HM. Hepatic abscesses in dogs: 14 cases (1982–1994). J Am Vet Med Assoc 1996; 208(2):243–247.
2. Sergeeff JS, Armstrong PJ, Bunch SE. Hepatic abscesses in cats: 14 cases (1985–2002). J Vet Intern Med 2004; 18:295–300.
3. Cotran RS, Kumar V, Collins T. Robbins: pathologic basis of disease. Philadelphia: WB Saunders Company; 2000.
4. Rubarth S. Leber und Gallenwege. In: Dobberstein J, Pallaske G, Stünzi H, eds. Joest - Handbuch der Speziellen Pathologischen Anatomie der Haustiere. 3rd edn. Berlin: Paul Parey Verlag; 1967:1–177.
5. Slappendel RJ, Ferrer L. Leishmaniasis. In: Greene CE, ed. Infectious diseases of the dog and cat. 2nd edn. Philadelphia: WB Saunders; 1998:450–458.
6. Kier AB, Greene CE. Cytauxzoonosis. In: Greene CE, ed. Infectious diseases of the dog and cat. 2nd edn. Philadelphia: WB Saunders; 1998:470–473.
7. Gillespie TN, Washabau RJ, Goldschmidt MH, et al. Detection of Bartonella henselae and Bartonella clarridgeiae DNA in hepatic specimens from two dogs with hepatic disease. J Am Vet Med Assoc 2003; 222(1):47–51, 35.
8. Greaves P. Histopathology of preclinical toxicity studies. 2nd edn. Amsterdam: Elsevier; 2000.
9. Greijdanus-van der Putten SWM, van Esch E, Kamerman J, et al. Drug/Induced protoporphyria in Beagle dogs-Toxicology Pathology; 2005; 33:720–725.
10. Veldhuis Kroeze EJ, Zentek J, Edixhoven-Bosdijk A, et al. Transient erythropoietic protoporphyria associated with chronic hepatitis and cirrhosis in a cohort of German shepherd dogs. Vet Rec 2006; 158:120–124.
11. Vatne M, Anderssson, M, Sevelius, E, et al. Immunohistochemical investigation of four glycoproteins in the hepatocytes of dogs with chronic liver disease. European J Vet Pathol 2001; 7:51–59.
12. Ossent P, Stockli RM, Pospischil A. Emperipolesis of lymphoid neoplastic cells in feline hepatocytes. Vet Pathol 1989; 26(3):279–280.
13. Jones TC, Hunt RD, King NW. Veterinary pathology. 6th edn. Baltimore: Williams and Wilkins; 1997.
14. Kelly WR. The liver and biliary system. In: Jubb KVF, Kennedy PC, Palmer N, eds. Pathology of domestic animals. 4th edn. San Diego: Academic Press; 1992:319–406.
15. Taylor RM, Farrow BR. Ceroid-lipofuscinosis in border collie dogs. Acta Neuropathol (Berl) 1988; 75(6):627–631.
16. Warren CD, Alroy J. Morphological, biochemical and molecular biology approaches for the diagnosis of lysosomal storage diseases. J Vet Diagn Invest 2000; 12(6):483–496.
17. Jolly RD, Walkley SU. Lysosomal storage diseases of animals: an essay in comparative pathology. Vet Pathol 1997; 34(6):527–548.
18. Nakayama H, Uchida K, Shouda T, et al. Systemic ceroid-lipofuscinosis in a Japanese domestic cat. J Vet Med Sci 1993; 55(5):829–831.
19. Hänichen T, Breuer W, Hermanns W. Canine lipid storage disease. Eur J Vet Path 1995; 1:37–44.
20. Keller CB, Lamarre J. Inherited lysosomal storage disease in an English springer spaniel. J Am Vet Med Assoc 1992; 200(2):194–195.
21. Herrtage ME, Palmer AC, Blakemore WF. Canine fucosidosis. Vet Rec 1985; 117(17):451–452.
22. Knowles K, Alroy J, Castagnaro M, et al. Adult-onset lysosomal storage disease in a Schipperke dog: clinical, morphological and biochemical studies. Acta Neuropathol (Berl) 1993; 86(3):306–312.
23. Muller G, Alldinger S, Moritz A, et al. GM1-gangliosidosis in Alaskan huskies: clinical and pathologic findings. Vet Pathol 2001; 38(3): 281–290.
24. Alroy J, Orgad U, Ucci AA, et al. Neurovisceral and skeletal GM1-gangliosidosis in dogs with beta-galactosidase deficiency. Science 1985; 229(4712):470–472.
25. Rodriguez M, O'Brien JS, Garrett RS, et al. Canine GM1 gangliosidosis. An ultrastructural and biochemical study. J Neuropathol Exp Neurol 1982; 41(6):618–629.
26. Saunders GK, Wood PA, Myers RK, et al. GM1 gangliosidosis in Portuguese water dogs: pathologic and biochemical findings. Vet Pathol 1988; 25(4):265–269.
27. Shell LG, Potthoff AI, Carithers R, et al. Neuronal-visceral GM1 gangliosidosis in Portuguese water dogs. J Vet Intern Med 1989; 3(1):1–7.
28. Yamato O, Ochiai K, Masuoka Y, et al. GM1 gangliosidosis in shiba dogs. Vet Rec 2000; 146(17):493–496.
29. De Maria R, Divari S, Bo S, et al. Beta-galactosidase deficiency in a Korat cat: a new form of feline GM1-gangliosidosis. Acta Neuropathol (Berl) 1998; 96(3):307–314.
30. Baker HJ, Walkley SU, Rattazzi MC, et al. Feline gangliosidoses as models of human lysosomal storage diseases. Prog Clin Biol Res 1982; 94:203–212.

31. Cummings JF, Wood PA, Walkley SU, et al. GM2 gangliosidosis in a Japanese spaniel. Acta Neuropathol (Berl) 1985; 67(3–4):247–253.

32. Yamato O, Matsuki N, Satoh H, et al. Sandhoff disease in a golden retriever dog. J Inherit Metab Dis 2002; 25(4):319–320.

33. Karbe E, Schiefer B. Familial amaurotic idiocy in male German Shorthair Pointers. Vet Pathol 1967; 6:223–232.

34. Cork LC, Munnell JF, Lorenz MD. The pathology of feline GM2 gangliosidosis. Am J Pathol 1978; 90(3):723–734.

35. Brix AE, Howerth EW, McConkie-Rosell A, et al. Glycogen storage disease type Ia in two littermate Maltese puppies. Vet Pathol 1995; 32(5): 460–465.

36. Ceh L, Hauge JG, Svenkerud R, et al. Glycogenosis type III in the dog. Acta Vet Scand 1976; 17(2):210–222.

37. Rafiquzzaman M, Svenkerud R, Strande A, et al. Glycogenosis in the dog. Acta Vet Scand 1976; 17:196–209.

38. Fyfe JC, Giger U, Van Winkle TJ, et al. Glycogen storage disease type iv: inherited deficiency of branching enzyme activity in cats. Pediatr Res 1992; 32:719–725.

39. Hartley WJ, Blakemore WF. Neurovisceral glucocerebroside storage (Gaucher's disease) in a dog. Vet Pathol 1973; 10(3):191–201.

40. Farrow BR, Hartley WJ, Pollard AC, et al. Gaucher disease in the dog. Prog Clin Biol Res 1982; 95:645–653.

41. Cummings JF, Wood PA, de Lahunta A, et al. The clinical and pathologic heterogeneity of feline alpha-mannosidosis. J Vet Intern Med 1988; 2(4):163–170.

42. Jezyk PF, Haskins ME, Newman LR. Alpha-mannosidosis in a Persian cat. J Am Vet Med Assoc 1986; 189(11):1483–1485.

43. Maenhout T, Kint JA, Dacremont G, et al. Mannosidosis in a litter of Persian cats. Vet Rec 1988; 122(15):351–354.

44. Hubler M, Haskins ME, Arnold S, et al. Mucolipidosis type II in a domestic shorthair cat. J Small Anim Pract 1996; 37(9):435–441.

45. Haskins ME, Otis EJ, Hayden JE, et al. Hepatic storage of glycosaminoglycans in feline and canine models of mucopolysaccharidoses I, VI, and VII. Vet Pathol 1992; 29(2):112–119.

46. Spellacy E, Shull RM, Constantopoulos G, et al. A canine model of human alpha-L-iduronidase deficiency. Proc Natl Acad Sci USA 1983; 80(19):6091–605.

47. Haskins ME, Aguirre GD, Jezyk PF, et al. The pathology of the feline model of mucopolysaccharidosis I. Am J Pathol 1983; 112(1):27–36.

48. Wilkerson MJ, Lewis DC, Marks SL, et al. Clinical and morphologic features of mucopolysaccharidosis type II in a dog: naturally occurring model of Hunter syndrome. Vet Pathol 1998; 35(3):230–233.

49. Fischer A, Carmichael KP, Munnell JF, et al. Sulfamidase deficiency in a family of Dachshunds: a canine model of mucopolysaccharidosis IIIA (Sanfilippo A). Pediatr Res 1998; 44(1):74–82.

50. Jolly RD, Ehrlich PC, Franklin RJ, et al. Histological diagnosis of mucopolysaccharidosis IIIA in a wire-haired dachshund. Vet Rec 2001; 148(18): 564–567.

51. Yogalingam G, Pollard T, Gliddon B, et al. Identification of a mutation causing mucopolysaccharidosis type IIIA in New Zealand Huntaway dogs. Genomics 2002; 79(2):150–153.

52. Neer TM, Dial SM, Pechman R, et al. Clinical vignette. Mucopolysaccharidosis VI in a miniature pinscher. J Vet Intern Med 1995; 9(6):429–433.

53. Haskins ME, Aguirre GD, Jezyk PF, et al. The pathology of the feline model of mucopolysaccharidosis VI. Am J Pathol 1980; 101(3):657–674.

54. Haskins ME, Aguirre GD, Jezyk PF, et al. Mucopolysaccharidosis type VII (Sly syndrome). Beta-glucuronidase-deficient mucopolysaccharidosis in the dog. Am J Pathol 1991; 138(6):1553–1555.

55. Schultheiss PC, Gardner SA, Owens JM, et al. Mucopolysaccharidosis VII in a cat. Vet Pathol 2000; 37(5):502–505.

56. Gitzelmann R, Bosshard NU, Superti-Furga A, et al. Feline mucopolysaccharidosis VII due to beta-glucuronidase deficiency. Vet Pathol 1994; 31(4):435–443.

57. Thompson JC, Johnstone AC, Jones BR, et al. The ultrastructural pathology of five lipoprotein lipase-deficient cats. J Comp Pathol 1989; 101(3): 251–262.

58. Johnstone AC, Jones BR, Thompson JC, et al. The pathology of an inherited hyperlipoproteinaemia of cats. J Comp Pathol 1990; 102(2):125–137.

59. Bundza A, Lowden JA, Charlton KM. Niemann-Pick disease in a poodle dog. Vet Pathol 1979; 16(5):530–538.

60. Kuwamura M, Awakura T, Shimada A, et al. Type C Niemann-Pick disease in a boxer dog. Acta Neuropathol (Berl) 1993; 85(3):345–348.

61. Lowenthal AC, Cummings JF, Wenger DA, et al. Feline sphingolipidosis resembling Niemann-Pick disease type C. Acta Neuropathol (Berl) 1990; 81(2):189–197.

62. Wenger DA, Sattler M, Kudoh T, et al. Niemann-Pick disease: a genetic model in Siamese cats. Science 1980; 208:1470–1473.

63. Mouwen JMVM, De Groot ECBM, eds. Atlas of veterinary pathology. Utrecht: Bunge; 1982.

Chapter **9**

Morphological classification of neoplastic disorders of the canine and feline liver

Jenny A. Charles, John M. Cullen, Ted S. G. A. M. van den Ingh, Tom Van Winkle, Valeer J. Desmet

INTRODUCTION

The neoplastic disorders of the liver in dogs and cats can be classified as:

1. Hepatocellular neoplasia, including nodular hyperplasia
2. Cholangiocellular neoplasia
3. Hepatic carcinoids and hepatoblastoma
4. Primary vascular and mesenchymal neoplasia
5. Hematopoietic neoplasia
6. Metastatic neoplasia.

HEPATOCELLULAR NEOPLASIA

Nodular hyperplasia

Nodular hyperplasia is a common disorder in older dogs but occurs less often in cats.[1,2] The incidence increases with age and almost all dogs over the age of 10 years show multiple hyperplastic nodules, which may range in size from 0.2 to 3.0 cm in diameter (Fig. 9.1). Histologically the lesion presents as a non-encapsulated nodule with a rather well-retained lobular arrangement, consisting of double-layered cords of well-differentiated hepatocytes and slight compression of the surrounding parenchyma (Fig. 9.2). Portal areas may be present within or at the periphery of the nodule, depending on the size of the nodular hyperplasia and its origin within the lobule. The nodules often show focal or diffuse lipidosis or glycogen accumulation of the hepatocytes. Nodular hyperplasia should be

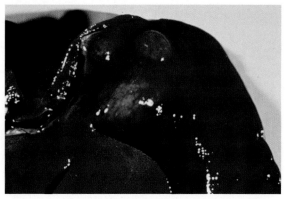

Figure 9.1 Dog. Nodular hyperplasia. (Reproduced from Mouwen JMVM, De Groot ECBM, eds. Atlas of veterinary pathology. Utrecht: Bunge; 1982, with permission).

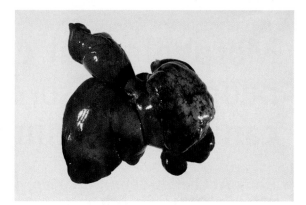

Figure 9.3 Cat. Hepatocellular adenoma.

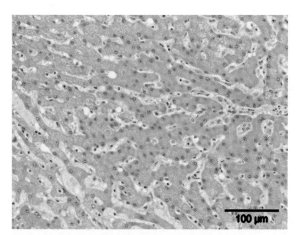

Figure 9.2 Dog. Nodular hyperplasia. Non-encapsulated nodule of double layered cords of hepatocytes. HE.

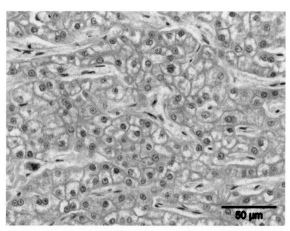

Figure 9.4 Dog. Hepatocellular adenoma. Trabeculae of well-differentiated hepatocytes with a uniform appearance. HE.

distinguished from regenerative nodules as seen in macronodular cirrhosis of the liver (see also Ch. 6 on parenchymal disorders). In macronodular cirrhosis, affected livers are grossly characterized by collapsed fibrotic areas and multiple nodules of varying size ranging from 0.2 cm to several centimeters in diameter.

Hepatocellular adenoma

Hepatocellular adenomas are seen in dogs[1-3] and cats.[1,4] In general they are restricted to one or two liver lobes and consist of friable pale tumors that closely resemble normal liver tissue (Fig. 9.3). His-

tologically, these are well-demarcated, mostly non-encapsulated hepatocellular tumors that lack portal tracts and bile ducts. They consist of cords or form trabeculae of well-differentiated hepatocytes (Fig. 9.4), separated by sometimes markedly dilated sinusoids and cystic blood and/or serum filled spaces. The hepatocytes have a uniform appearance and the nuclei are similar to those in normal hepatocytes, but nucleoli may be more prominent. Mitotic figures are rare. Often focal or more extensive areas with macrovesicular or mixed type lipidosis or marked glycogen accumulation of the neoplastic hepatocytes are observed. Sometimes foci of extramedullary hemopoiesis and Fe-pigment containing macrophages can be seen.

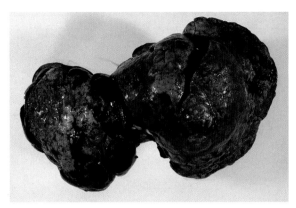

Figure 9.5   Dog. Hepatocellular carcinoma.

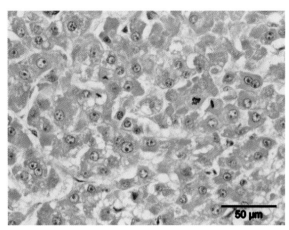

Figure 9.6   Dog. Hepatocellular carcinoma. Trabeculae of hepatocytes with cellular pleiomorphism and multiple mitotic figures. HE.

Hepatocellular carcinoma

Hepatocellular carcinomas are malignant neoplasms of hepatocytes and are infrequently seen in both dogs[1–3,5,6] and cats.[1,2,7] They may occur as large solitary structures that resemble normal liver tissue, but also may be seen widespread throughout the liver (Fig. 9.5). Metastases occur within the liver and to the regional (hepatic) lymph nodes, but distant metastases can also be found. Histologically they form irregular trabeculae separated by sometimes markedly dilated sinusoids and cystic blood and/or serum filled spaces, or form acinar or large solid structures. The cytological features of the hepatocytes in hepatocellular carcinomas are variable; they may be rather well differentiated or very poorly differentiated. They can be differentiated from hepatocellular adenomas by: infiltrative growth at the periphery of the tumor, by regional or diffuse presence of cellular pleiomorphism, sometimes with atypical or bizarre cells and sometimes even atypical multinucleated cells; variation in cell and nuclear size; one or multiple nucleoli of varying size; and by the frequent presence of mitotic figures (Figs 9.6, 9.7). Often, focal or widespread lipidosis or glycogen accumulation of the neoplastic hepatocytes are observed. Sometimes foci of extramedullary hemopoiesis and Fe-pigment containing macrophages can be seen.

Both hepatocellular carcinomas and adenomas may develop extensive central necrosis, which may develop secondary abscesses (see also Ch. 8).

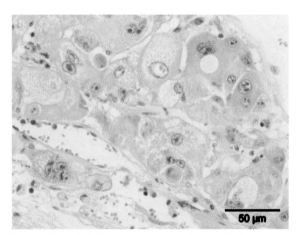

Figure 9.7   Cat. Hepatocellular carcinoma. Trabeculae of atypical, bizarre and multinucleated hepatocytes. HE.

CHOLANGIOCELLULAR NEOPLASIA

Cholangiocellular adenoma (biliary adenoma)

Cholangiocellular adenomas are solitary, well-circumscribed tumors and are extremely rare in both dogs and cats.[1,2] They show expansive growth and consist of slightly dilated, occasionally cystic structures, lined with cuboidal or flattened, well-differentiated biliary epithelium. They should be differentiated from unilocular or multilocular cysts or Von Meyenburg complexes as seen in congenital cystic diseases of the liver (see also Ch. 5 on

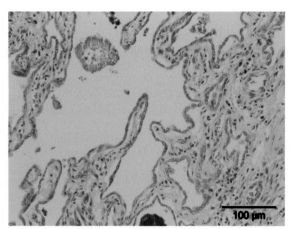

Figure 9.8   Dog. Adult polycystic disease. Irregularly formed bile ducts with cystic dilatation. HE.

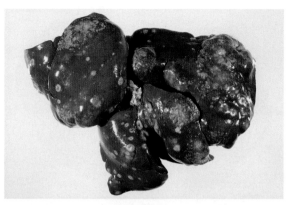

Figure 9.9   Dog. Cholangiocellular carcinoma. Multiple irregularly formed tumors, often showing central umbilication.

biliary disorders) These cystic lesions (which are often mistaken for cholangiocellular adenomas) typically show irregular cystic spaces lined with cuboidal to flattened epithelium (Fig. 9.8), varying amounts of fibrous tissue, and often islands of hepatocytes that are interspersed between the cysts.

Cholangiocellular carcinoma (biliary carcinoma)

Cholangiocellular carcinomas are malignant neoplasms of biliary epithelium and usually arise from the intrahepatic bile ducts. They are seen in both dogs and cats[1–3,6,7] and may occur as a large single mass, but often present as multiple irregularly formed tumors. They have a whitish appearance and firm consistency, and often show central umbilication (Fig. 9.9). Microscopically they have an acinar, ductular and/or papillary growth pattern (Fig. 9.10) and are often associated with marked fibroplasia (Fig. 9.11). In well-differentiated areas, mucin may be detected in the lumen of these structures. The differentiation of the neoplastic cells varies and usually there is marked pleiomorphism and mitotic figures are regularly encountered. The margins of the tumor clearly show invasion of tumor cells in the surrounding parenchyma. Spread within the liver particularly results from metastases along the portal lymphatics and the portal vein (Fig. 9.12). Metastases to the regional (hepatic) lymph nodes, as well as distant metastases, are fre-

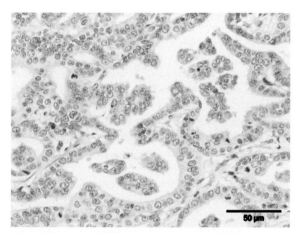

Figure 9.10   Dog. Cholangiocellular carcinoma. Papillary growth of rather well-differentiated bile duct epithelium with multiple mitotic figures. HE.

quently seen. Cholangiocellular carcinomas may also arise from the extrahepatic bile ducts and, apart from metastases, may cause obstruction of the common bile duct and thus extrahepatic cholestasis. In cats, chronic cholangitis due to liver fluke infestation has been associated with the development of intrahepatic and extrahepatic cholangiocellular carcinomas.[8]

Mixed hepatocellular and cholangiocellular carcinomas

Sometimes primary hepatic tumors with a mixed histological pattern of hepatocellular differentia-

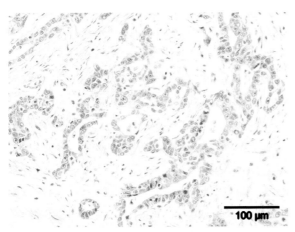

Figure 9.11 Dog. Cholangiocellular carcinoma. Papillary growth of pleiomorphic bile duct epithelium with marked fibroplasias. HE.

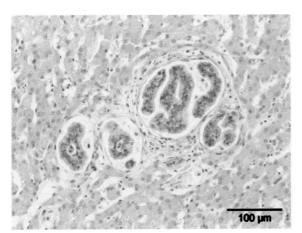

Figure 9.12 Dog. Cholangiocellular carcinoma. Intrahepatic metastases often occur along the portal vein and lymphatics. HE.

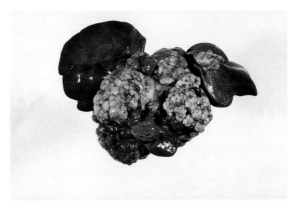

Figure 9.13 Cat. Hepatic carcinoid.

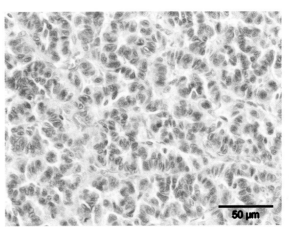

Figure 9.14 Cat. Hepatic carcinoid; ribbon type pattern. HE.

tion and cholangiocellular differentiation are observed.[3]

Immunohistochemical staining may be helpful in the classification of primary epithelial tumors of the liver. In formalin-fixed, paraffin-embedded material, hepatocellular tumors stain positive with few exceptions, with the monoclonal antibody hepatocyte paraffin 1 (HepPar1), whereas cholangiocellular tumors stain positive with few exceptions, with a monoclonal antibody to cytokeratin 7 (CK 7); a single hepatocellular carcinoma has been studied that contained cells positive for both HepPar1 and CK7 suggesting the presence of intermediate cells within the tumor.[9]

HEPATIC CARCINOID AND HEPATOBLASTOMA

Hepatic carcinoids are rare neoplasms in dogs[1,10] and cats.[1,7,11] Carcinoids can be recognized in both intrahepatic and extrahepatic sites. They can form solitary masses (Fig. 9.13) but, particularly in intrahepatic tumors, they can also occur as multiple nodules, probably owing to intrahepatic metastasis. Histologically, hepatic carcinoids are characterized by cells organized in rosettes, cords or ribbons (Figs 9.14, 9.15). Cells may be small, elongated or

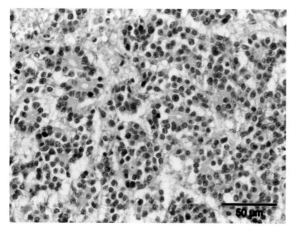

Figure 9.15   Dog. Hepatic carcinoid; rosette type pattern. HE.

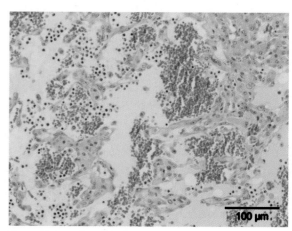

Figure 9.16   Dog. Hemangiosarcoma. HE.

fusiform and darkly stained with hyperchromatic nuclei and little cytoplasm, or they may be polygonal and relatively large with round to oval hyperchromatic nuclei and pale or granular cytoplasm; mitotic figures are regularly seen. The diagnosis of hepatic carcinoid is based on positive staining of the neoplastic cells for neuroendocrine cell markers like chromogranin A and neuron-specific enolase or the presence of neurosecretory granules with electron microscopy.

Hepatic carcinoids are thought to originate from pre-existing neuroendocrine cells in the epithelium of the intrahepatic and extrahepatic bile ducts and the gall bladder, but they may also possibly arise from hepatic progenitor cells as these also show morphological characteristics of neuroendocrine cells. Hepatic progenitor cells (oval cells) are small cells with round to oval hyperchromatic nuclei, which stain, at least in humankind, positive for several neuroendocrine markers.[12]

Hepatoblastomas, which frequently occur in children and are thought to arise from hepatic progenitor cells, also show positive staining of the neoplastic cells for various neuroendocrine cell markers like S100, chromogranin A and neuron-specific enolase.[13] Hepatoblastomas have been described in domestic animals such as lambs[14] and in a foal[15] but until now have not been recognized in dogs and cats.

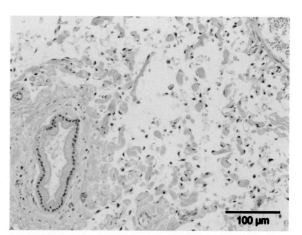

Figure 9.17   Dog. Lymphangiosarcoma; extension in the portal area. HE.

PRIMARY VASCULAR AND MESENCHYMAL NEOPLASIA

Primary vascular and mesenchymal tumors, except for hemangiosarcoma, are extremely rare in dogs and cats.[1] Apart from the already mentioned hemangiosarcoma (Fig. 9.16), they include lymphangioma, lymphangiosarcoma (Fig. 9.17), fibrosarcoma, leiomyosarcoma, malignant mesenchymoma, osteosarcoma and rhabdomyosarcoma. These tumors have the same gross and histological characteristics as those that arise at other more commonly affected sites of the body.

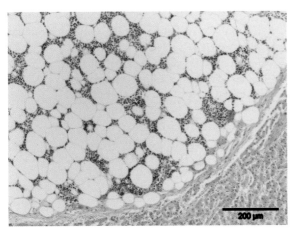

Figure 9.18   Cat. Myelolipoma. HE.

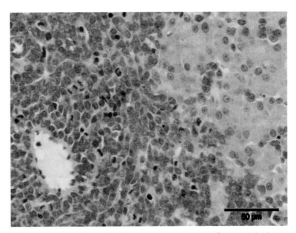

Figure 9.19   Dog. Malignant lymphoma. Centrolobular area. HE.

Myelolipoma

Myelolipoma of the liver is a very rare benign tumor or tumor-like lesion and has only been reported in cats and wild felids.[1,2] They are usually found as multiple growths that may be located in more than one lobe of the liver. Myelolipomas are rather well-delineated or surrounded by a thin capsule and are composed of mature and normal appearing adipose and myeloid tissue resembling normal bone marrow (Fig. 9.18).

HEMATOPOIETIC NEOPLASIA

The liver is often involved in hemotopoietic neoplasia, usually as part of generalized or visceral forms of the disease. The organ is usually affected diffusely and has a swollen, pale appearance, often with a zonal (lobular) pattern, but nodular infiltration can also occur.

Malignant lymphoma is the most frequent type observed and, histologically, often shows particular involvement of the portal areas and the connective tissue around the hepatic veins (Fig. 9.19). Both B- and T-cell malignant lymphomas are seen. Rarely, an epitheliotropic variant of T-cell malignant lymphoma is observed with marked emperipolesis of the tumor cells by the hepatocytes (Fig. 9.20).[16]

Other types of hematopoietic neoplasms involving the liver include the whole spectrum of

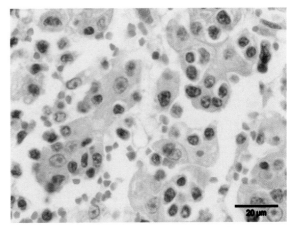

Figure 9.20   Cat. Epitheliotropic malignant lymphoma with emperipolesis of neoplastic lymphocytes by hepatocytes. HE.

hematopoietic cells and include erythremic myelosis, systemic and malignant histiocytosis, mast cell leucosis (malignant mastocytosis), megakaryocytic leucosis, neutrophilic, eosinophilic and basophilic myeloid leucosis, monocytic leucosis, and plasma cell leucosis.

METASTATIC NEOPLASIA

Metastatic neoplasia in the liver of the dog and cat is more common than primary neoplasia. They usually occur as multiple neoplastic foci of different size and, histologically, they resemble the primary tumor.

SUMMARY

Neoplastic disorders of the liver are classified as:

1. Hepatocellular neoplasia including nodular hyperplasia, hepatocellular adenoma and hepatocellular carcinoma
2. Cholangiocellular neoplasia including cholangiocellular adenoma and cholangiocellular carcinoma
3. Hepatic carcinoids and hepatoblastoma
4. Primary vascular and mesenchymal neoplasia of the liver
5. Hematopoietic neoplasia
6. Metastatic neoplasia.

References

1. Cullen JM, Popp JA. Tumors of the liver and gall bladder. In: Meuten DJ, ed. Tumors in Domestic Animals. 4th edn. Ames: Iowa State Press; 2002:483–508.
2. Kelly WR. The liver and biliary system. In: Jubb KVF, Kennedy PC, Palmer N, eds. Pathology of domestic animals. 4th edn. San Diego: Academic Press; 1992:319–406.
3. Trigo FJ, Thompson H, Breeze RG, et al. The pathology of liver tumours in the dog. J Comp Pathol 1982; 92(1):21–39.
4. Lawrence HJ, Erb HN, Harvey HJ. Nonlymphomatous hepatobiliary masses in cats: 41 cases (1972 to 1991). Vet Surg 1994; 23(5):365–368.
5. Patnaik AK, Hurvitz AI, Lieberman PH, et al. Canine hepatocellular carcinoma. Vet Pathol 1981; 18(4):427–438.
6. Patnaik AK, Hurvitz AI, Lieberman PH. Canine hepatic neoplasms: a clinicopathologic study. Vet Pathol 1980; 17(5):553–564.
7. Patnaik AK. A morphologic and immunocytochemical study of hepatic neoplasms in cats. Vet Pathol 1992; 29(5):405–415.
8. Wetzel R. Parasitäre Erkrankungen der Leber und der Gallenwege. In: Dobberstein J, Pallaske G, Stünzi H, eds. Joest – Handbuch der Speziellen Pathologischen Anatomie der Haustiere. 3rd edn. Berlin: Paul Parey Verlag; 1967:209–299.
9. Ramos-Vara JA, Miller MA, Johnson GC. Immunohistochemical characterization of canine hyperplastic hepatic lesions and hepatocellular and biliary neoplasms with monoclonal antibody hepatocyte paraffin 1 and a monoclonal antibody to cytokeratin 7. Vet Pathol 2001; 38(6):636–643.
10. Patnaik AK, Lieberman PH, Hurvitz AI, et al. Canine hepatic carcinoids. Vet Pathol 1981; 18(4):445–453.
11. Alexander RW, Kock RA. Primary hepatic carcinoid (APUD cell carcinoma) in the cat. J Small Anim Pract 1982; 23:767–771.
12. Roskams T, De Vos R, Van den Oord JJ, et al. Cells with neuroendocrine features in regenerating human liver. Apmis 1991; 23(Suppl):32–39.
13. Anthony PP. Tumours and tumour-like lesions of the liver and biliary tract: aetiology, epidemiology and pathology. In: McSween RNM, Burt AD, Portmann BC, eds. Pathology of the Liver. 4th edn. London: Churchill Livingstone; 2002:711–775.
14. Manktelow BW. Hepatoblastomas in sheep. J Pathol Bact 1965; 89:711–714.
15. Neu SM. Hepatoblastoma in an equine fetus. J Vet Diagn Invest 1993; 5:634–637.
16. Ossent P, Stockli RM, Pospischil A. Emperipolesis of lymphoid neoplastic cells in feline hepatocytes. Vet Pathol 1989; 26(3):279–280.
17. Mouwen JMVM, De Groot ECBM, eds. Atlas of veterinary pathology. Utrecht: Bunge; 1982.

Subject Index